Thoracoscopic Repair of Esophageal Atresia

Ravi P Kanojia

Thoracoscopic Repair of Esophageal Atresia

Springer

Ravi P Kanojia
Professor, Pediatric Surgery
Chandigarh, Punjab, India

ISBN 978-981-97-5694-0 ISBN 978-981-97-5695-7 (eBook)
https://doi.org/10.1007/978-981-97-5695-7

This Springer imprint is published by the registered company Springer Nature Singapore Pte Ltd.
The registered company address is: 152 Beach Road, #21-01/04 Gateway East, Singapore 189721, Singapore

Dedicated to my grandfather, Shri Ram Prasad Kanojia. He was a beacon of wisdom, strength, and vision for family. His gentle guidance shaped the person I am today. As I navigate the pages of life, I carry with me the strength of his character. This dedication is a humble tribute to his life and remarkable soul whose presence will forever resonate in my life.

Ravi P Kanojia

Foreword

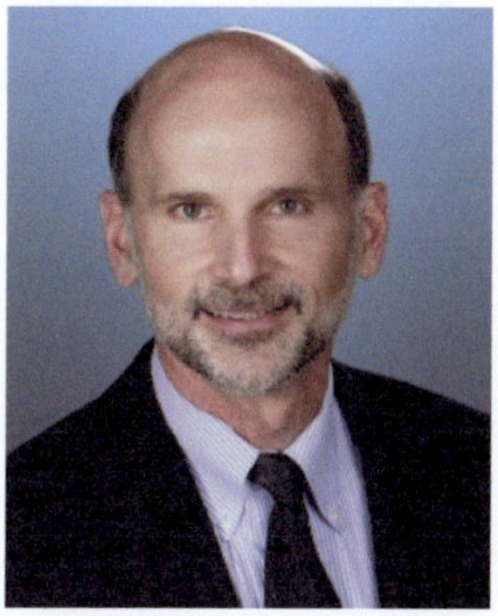

As pediatric surgeons, we must not only deal with complex congenital anomalies but we must think about and treat the consequences of the procedures we perform. To this end there is no more morbid incision performed by pediatric surgeons than that of a thoracotomy in a newborn infant. The incidence of scoliosis, shoulder girdle weakness, and chest wall deformity following thoracotomy is as high as 40%. There are also new studies with rapid sequence MRI which show significant lung and chest wall restriction and asymmetry in children who had a thoracotomy for trachea-esophageal atresia (TEF) or congenital pulmonary airway malformation (CPAM) as an infant.

For this reason, it is beholden on those of us to treat infants to eliminate this morbidity wherever possible.

In 1999, Dr. Tom Lobe and I performed the first thoracoscopic repair of a pure esophageal atresia (EA) in Berlin during the International Pediatric Endosurgery Group (IPEG) meeting. One year later I performed the first thoracoscopic repair of an EA and TEF in a healthy 3.2 kg newborn in Denver, Colorado. Since that time, we have performed all of our TEFs this way. This has allowed us to avoid the complications of a large thoracic incision. We also feel we perform the procedure with more precision because we see the anatomy much better because of the magnified view.

But this is a technically demanding procedure and requires a new skill set of advanced minimally invasive surgery (MIS) skills. Twenty-five years after completion of the first thoracoscopic TEF in Denver, less than 25% of the TEFs done in the United States are approached thoracoscopically, meaning the majority of patients are still getting a thoracotomy.

Given the major advantages of high-tech equipment and resources available in the United States, and the low adoption rate, this makes this book by Dr. Ravi Kanojia all the more impressive.

I have had the honor of visiting India to operate and teach on a number of occasions, and each time I was amazed at the skill level of the surgeons and their ability to do more with less. I met Dr. Kanojia a number of years ago in India at one of their national congresses, when he presented a video on the thoracoscopic repair of TEF, and won an award for it.

This book is a testament to the skill and commitment of Dr. Kanojia and his colleagues, and his desire to share his experience and technical knowledge with his colleagues in India and around the world.

It is my pleasure to congratulate him on his clinical work and this book on the thoracoscopic repair of EA/TEF, something I have spent a large part of my career trying to refine and teach to others.

Rocky Mountain Hospital for Children
Denver, CO, USA

Steven S. Rothenberg

Preface

Esophageal atresia is a challenging anomaly for Pediatric Surgeons. The understanding of the science of this condition has evolved over two centuries. In the modern era, survival has universally become an expectant outcome for neonates born with this condition. Plenty of literature is available to help understand esophageal atresia and its treatment. Minimal access treatment of this condition is a two-and-a-half decade-old procedure, and outcomes have significantly improved with this new approach. Thoracoscopic repair of esophageal atresia (TREAT) is a technically demanding procedure with less margin of safety and error. There is significantly less fragmented information present in literature if a beginner has to educate himself about minor details on this delicate operation. This book covers all aspects of TREAT. The book explains the entire procedure, from the anatomy, setup, anesthesia, surgery steps, and various anatomical issues with different patients. It also presents a review of the evidence in the literature. The chapters provide a systematic approach for anyone learning this procedure with extensive pictorial depiction. The book aims to be a one-stop guide and reference for anyone wanting to perform TREAT.

I thank the co-authors listed, who contributed some of the specialty chapters on anesthesia.

Writing this book has been a journey of learning for me. It has made me realize how little I know and that there is so much to learn.

Chandigarh, Punjab, India — Ravi P. Kanojia

Acknowledgment

I sincerely thank Prof. Neerja Bharadwaj and Dr. Aditi Jain for contributing Chap. 4 on anesthesia and ventilation and Chap. 14. They have brought unique expertise and insights that enriched the contents of this book. Their contribution is invaluable and provides completeness to the subject matter. I also thank Prof V Raveenthiran for reviewing chapter 1 on history of esophageal atresia surgery. His valuable inputs made the chapter better.

About This Book

Esophageal atresia is a common neonatal emergency, and surgical repair in the newborn period is conventionally achieved by thoracotomy. With the development in pediatric minimal access surgery, esophageal atresia repair has been done with thoracoscopy after its first description in 1999. Many centers now prefer the thoracoscopic approach, which is claimed to be beneficial in terms of outcome both in the short and long term. Neonatal thoracoscopy is a difficult procedure and has a long learning curve. It requires a team approach with a competent anesthetist and surgical assistant. A surgeon alone cannot accomplish this procedure. This book presents comprehensive details on the procedure of thoracoscopic repair of esophageal atresia. The chapters sequentially explain all the procedure steps, from setup, instrumentation, patient selection, and ergonomics to detailed stepwise descriptions of the operative procedure. Since esophageal atresia can have so many variations in anatomy, the chapters cover how to tackle these variations. To keep the reader's interest, a detailed review of history and current literature, along with controversies, is presented. Interested readers will start from the history as the first chapter and can go through the descriptions of the entire procedure from start to finish. Any pediatric surgery trainee interested in pediatric minimal access discipline will find this book as a one-stop resource on everything they want to know about thoracoscopic repair of esophageal atresia. This book also includes coverage of nonsurgical aspects such as anesthesia and ventilation and effects on cerebral oxygenation during thoracoscopy. The book presents topics in easy-to-understand English and is richly supplemented with illustrations and high-resolution operative photographs. Video clips also supplement the text wherever an operative step is explained. These videos are linked to the publisher's website for easy access.

Contents

Thoroscopic Repair of Esophageal Atresia and Tracheoesophageal Fistula (TREAT): A Brief Introduction to the Current State of the Art and Surgical History

1

Contents

Learning Objectives

1. Introduction to the procedure of TREAT
2. Historical phases in the evolution of esophageal atresia surgery
3. Evolution of surgical procedures for esophageal atresia

1.1 Introduction

Esophageal atresia is the most common congenital anomaly of the esophagus and is the third commonest congenital anomaly of newborns, with the incidence of 1 in 3000–4000 live births [1]. In the Indian subcontinent, it is a common newborn pediatric surgical emergency. There has been a paradigm shift in the survival of newborns with esophageal atresia. The development of diagnostic techniques, anesthesia, and multi-disciplinary neonatal care has brought a revolutionary change with increasing survival in both syndromic and isolated cases [2, 3]. This, however, was not the case historically. Esophageal atresia surgery has evolved over a period of

R. P. Kanojia, *Thoracoscopic Repair of Esophageal Atresia*,
https://doi.org/10.1007/978-981-97-5695-7_1

three centuries since its first recognition in 1670. The history period from 1670 to the current day and age has seen 0% survival except for the last 90 years. It took a significant length of time to understand the anomaly, and with the continued development of neonatal surgical care, survival became a reality. There has been exponential development in the science of esophageal atresia management, and it has reached the highest level of sophistication with thoracoscopy and minimally invasive repair. This chapter describes the chronology and history of the development of esophageal atresia surgery leading to current practices.

1.2 History

Delving through the evolution of esophageal atresia surgery, the timeline can be divided into four phases: first is the 1670–1913 Phase I, when the first ever discoveries were made, as mentioned in the following sections; second is Phase II, 1913–1960, the era of anatomical understanding and the first successful survival of esophageal atresia neonate. This was followed by Phase III from 1960 to 1999, the era led by Ladd, Lanmann, and Haight, who pioneered the surgical procedure and reported survival with many others and made survival an expectant outcome in esophageal atresia. Phase IV runs from 1999 till the current day, the phase of sophistication with modern anesthesia, ventilation, intensive care, and minimally invasive surgery with nearly 100% expectant outcome.

1.2.1 Phase I: 1670–1913

Historically first descriptions of esophageal atresia date to 1670 [4]. This was a description of a discontinuous esophagus in a conjoint twin with the esophagus of the right twin being described as “not open as it was probed” and discontinuity checked with blowing wind (Fig. 1.1). This was published in Philosophical Transactions of the Royal Society, in the same year. In this publication detailed description was presented for the anatomical features of the unseparated conjoint twins, and the esophagus was described as non-continuous in one of the twins. The term esophageal atresia was not used at that time. The first case of esophageal atresia with tracheoesophageal fistula was recognized and published by Thomas Gibson in 1697 [5]. He described the condition in his book *Anatomy of Human Body Epitomized.* Till this time there was no proper understanding of the types of esophageal atresia, i.e., with fistula and without fistula and the condition was uniformly fatal. This went on for a long period with no published information until 1839 when Thomas Hill [6] described an infant with the inability to swallow and had aspirated and choked on feeding. He thought that there could be some sort of esophageal spasm and that stimulating the rectum can give some relief, only to find out that the child had no rectum either. This is the first known case of esophageal atresia with associated anomaly of anorectal malformation. After this Harold Hirschsprung described ten cases in 1861 [7] followed by Mackenzie documenting 37 cases in 1880 [8].

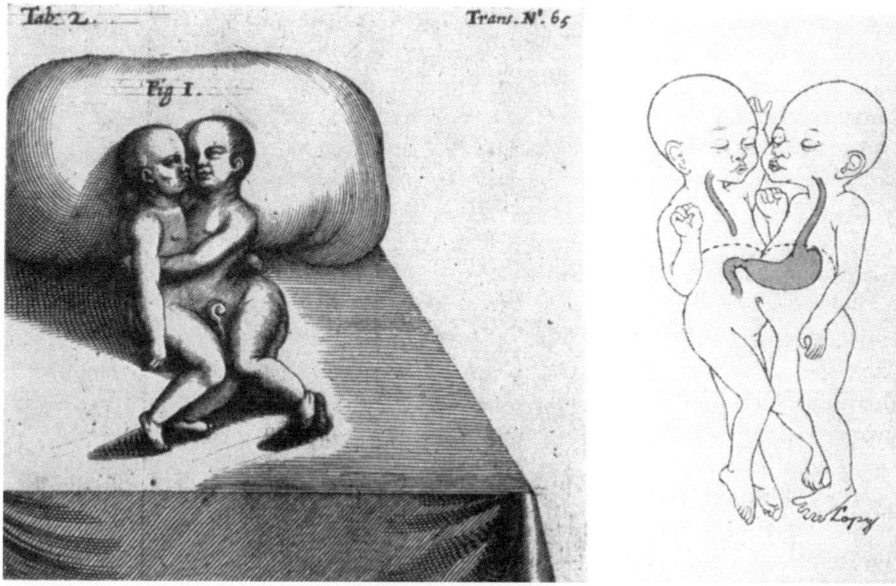

Fig. 1.1 Original illustration from the Philosophical Transactions of Royal Society reporting esophageal atresia in one of the conjoint twins. (Reproduced with permission)

There is no published description after this until the next phase, as no one took interest due to fatality, and the incidence of the condition was very low or not diagnosed.

1.2.2 Phase II: 1913–1939

In 1913 a pediatrician, Joseph B [9], described two cases where feeding jejunostomy and gastrostomy was done in each of these two cases. These two patients still died due to aspiration as nothing was done to the upper pouch. In the same year, Richter H [10] identified thoracotomy as the treatment for correction of discontinuous esophagus. He wrote that the anatomy of the neonatal chest is complex, and the small structures are difficult to deal with. His patients survived for few hours after surgery. This was the phase when it was recognized that esophageal atresia can have many variants and requires opening of the chest. However, opening the chest and ventilating a child were a huge challenge which made surgeons think if the problem can be handled via the abdomen which is a much easier approach and the child is easy to ventilate. In 1936 Gage M and Oschner A [11] did ligation of the esophagus at the level of the gastric cardia. This is the primitive form of fistula ligation that we do today at the level of the trachea. Some surgeons made two gastrostomies one as proximal to decompress the tracheoesophageal fistula and second distally for feeding. All these described patients died. These surgeons were although technically unsuccessful but were on the right path to understand that the correct treatment of this condition is to ligate the fistula communication and do end-to-end esophageal anastomosis. Charles Mixter (in 1929) and Thomas Lanmann (in 1933) [12] recognized that posterior extra-pleural approach is the correct method which stands till date. Lanmann was the first person to do an end-to-end anastomosis in his two patients, but his patients also died within 3 h after surgery. This reflected that the procedure was too extensive at that time, especially in an era when anesthesia technique was still evolving.

1.2.3 Phase III: 1939–1999

The learnings of surgeons in Phase II had set the technical ground for surgeons like Ladd and Cameroon Haight. They knew what needed to be done, and they had to just figure out how to achieve the intrathoracic procedure with proper ventilation and anesthesia.

William Ladd in 1939 [13] treated a baby with esophageal atresia with tracheo-esophageal fistula. Instead of going for thoracotomy, he did gastrostomy on the second day of birth and aspirated the upper pouch repeatedly with nursing care. The baby survived for 4 months. He later did a cervical esophagostomy to prevent aspiration. This patient survived and did well. Ladd then went on to do an esophageal replacement operation where he made a skin-lined tube which drained with gravity. He called this operation esophageal marsupialization. This patient was a girl born on 29 November 1939 and was the first longest surviving patient of esophageal atresia with treatment done. He identified the fact that the respiratory tract needs to be protected early in life. From 1941 to 1942, he operated six more patients. He finally published in 1944 with 15 cases and had 9 survivors with a survival percentage of 60% [13]. This was a significant improvement and paradigm shift from 0% before 1939 to 60% within 3 years. His operation did not involve primary anastomosis of esophagus which was later improved upon by Cameroon Haight.

Haight in 1941 reported a successful outcome with a series of patients with patients surviving to be alive till adulthood. The case description of the first baby done by Cameroon Haight is very interesting [14]. He was referred to a baby of esophageal atresia who had survived till day 8 without much sickness and respiratory complications. The baby had a 500-mile trip from another city to Ann Arbor and survived the trip. On arrival baby was 3.66 kg and was quite well because of which Haight agreed to accept the baby for correction. He did a left thoracotomy on 15 March 1941. Open drop anesthesia method was used for inducing the baby, and a tight face mask was placed for ventilation. The thoracotomy involved removing four centimeters of second to fifth posterior ribs to gain exposure. Since he was on the left side, he had to mobilize the great vessels. He performed a single-layer anastomosis and closed the chest with a rubber drain. The baby survived the operation and did well. The anastomosis leaked, and there was saliva from the chest wound. Following this he did a gastrostomy. Haight even tried to pass a rubber catheter trans-anastomotic so that he can use it for stenting and feeding. But during this attempt, the tube came out through the chest wound. This leak however gradually settled, and the baby started taking oral feedings and later gastrostomy was removed. Haight then did esophageal dilatation at the age of 17 months.

He presented this patient as the sole surviving patient in a series of 15 babies. This success led to many referrals coming to Haight. In 1944 Haight presented his total experience of 32 cases with 6 survivors. It is interesting to know that Haight was using the left posterolateral approach for anastomosis until his 11th case when he recognized that the same thing can be done much more easily from right approach avoiding the mobilization of aorta. After this right posterolateral thoracotomy was the standard approach which stands correct till today.

After this several series reported more than 50% survival [15] with Waterston reporting 57% survival [16]. A series by Swenson and Ladd reported 37% survival with a staged approach and 44% survival with primary anastomosis [17]. There has been exponential improvement in techniques and management with more than 90% survival in the 1990s. The descendants of Cameroon Haight who were Arnold Coran, Peter Manning, and Herbert Sloan reported 83% survival in 1986 [18].

The clear understanding of technicalities, better support of anesthesia and use of antimicrobials, and the developing field of minimal invasive surgery pushed surgeons to approach this condition from a keyhole surgery perspective which heralds the next era in the development of esophageal atresia surgery.

1.2.4 Phase IV: 1999–2023

With the development of anesthesia and neonatal care, we have come a long way with the minimal access approach to esophageal atresia. The first case done by thoracoscopic approach was by T Lobe and S Rothenberg, and this case was done just before an international pediatric endosurgery group (IPEG) meeting in Berlin. The patient was a 2-month-old baby with pure esophageal atresia who was initially managed by esophageal bouginage for lengthening. They used a 3-trocar approach and used a bronchial blocker to control the right lung and did extra-corporeal knotting to do the esophageal anastomosis [19].

This was followed by S. Rothenberg a year later in 2000 reporting a successful treatment of esophageal atresia with fistula by thoracoscopic approach [20]. He concluded that thoracoscopic repair may become routine although the procedure presents formidable technical challenges. Since then, thoracoscopic repair adoption has been widespread, and majority of the advanced centers have reported successful outcome. The first largest series of 100 cases spread across multi-institution was reported by Holcomb in 2003 [21]. Chapter 11 presents a summation of 6 systematic review and meta-analysis collating data of more than 1500 patients to draw conclusions that thoracoscopic repair is equally good with open repair and even offers several advantages over the morbid chest opening approach.

Figure 1.2 is an infographic summarizing the timeline for the development of esophageal atresia surgery leading to the current practices. It shows 1939 as the watershed line when the era changed from zero survival to >50% survival in the 1940s and 1950s.

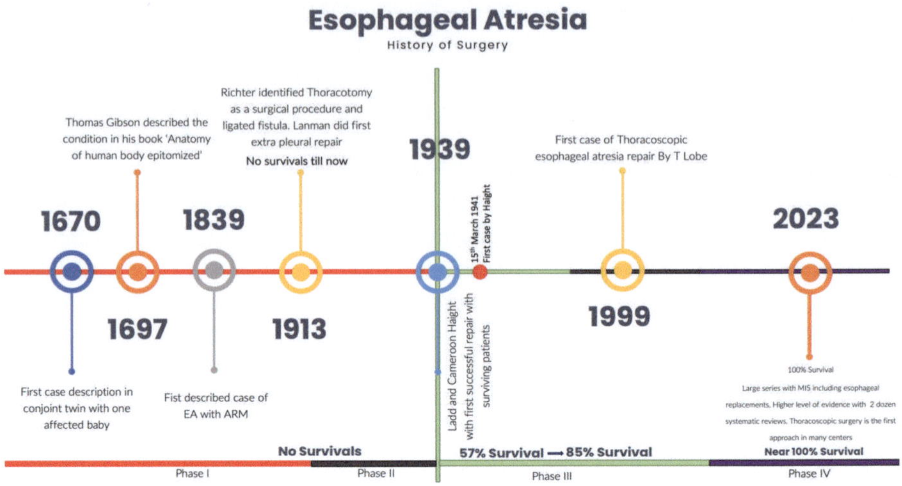

Fig. 1.2 Infographic summarizing the timeline for the development of esophageal atresia surgery leading to the current practices

1.3 Evolution of Surgical Operations for Esophageal Atresia

After the first description in 1670, it was not until 1913 that the first description of any attempt for esophageal atresia surgery was seen. The early attempts of saving neonates were in the form of gastrostomy. Richter in the same year did a posterior thoracotomy. Charles Mixter in 1929 was the first to do a thoracotomy with an extra-pleural approach. He did fistula ligation with dorsal esophagostomy. Lanmann was the first to perform a primary esophageal anastomosis via thoracotomy, but none of his patients survived. William Ladd in 1939 was the first to have a survivor of esophageal atresia described in the Phase III section above. This was followed by Cameroon Haight having a first survivor after a primary esophageal anastomosis. Haight gets most of the credit for this even though Lanmann had done a similar procedure before, but none of his patients survived. After this thoracotomy and primary anastomosis become the standard operation for classic variety of esophageal atresia. As the neonatal science evolved, the thoracoscopic approach was first done in 1999. Figure 1.3 is an infographic representing the evolution of the surgical operations documented in history for esophageal atresia.

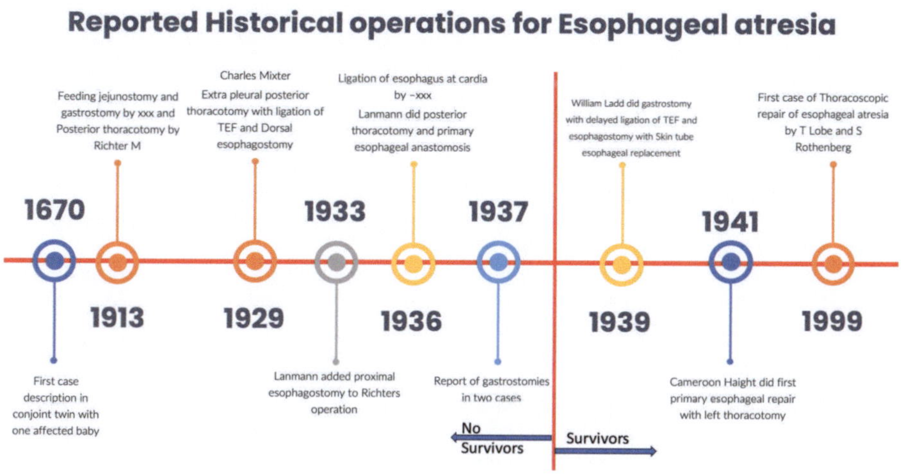
Reported Historical operations for Esophageal atresia
1670
First case description in conjoint twin with one affected baby
Feeding jejunostomy and gastrostomy by xxx and Posterior thoracotomy by Richter M
1913
Charles Mixter Extra pleural posterior thoracotomy with ligation of TEF and Dorsal esophagostomy
1929
1933
Lanmann added proximal esophagostomy to Richters operation
Ligation of esophagus at cardia by -xxx Lanmann did posterior thoracotomy and primary esophageal anastomosis
1936
1937
Report of gastrostomies in two cases
No Survivors
Survivors
William Ladd did gastrostomy with delayed ligation of TEF and esophagostomy with Skin tube esophageal replacement
1939
1941
Cameroon Haight did first primary esophageal repair with left thoracotomy
First case of Thoracoscopic repair of esophageal atresia by T Lobe and S Rothenberg
1999

Fig. 1.3 Infographic representing the evolution of the surgical operations documented in history for esophageal atresia

1.4 Current Status and Acceptance of Thoracoscopy

Thoracoscopic repair since 1999 is now in two-and-a-half-decade-old procedure, and the adoption of the procedure is widespread with significant success in many centers. Chapter 12 deals with the literature review which lists several meta-analyses done for comparison of open versus thoracoscopic repair. The current data is sufficient to prove the feasibility of the procedure, and it goes beyond to show that it is very much comparable to open procedure in every aspect, be it the intraoperative parameters or long-term outcomes and complications.

1.5 Conclusions

To conclude esophageal atresia management has come a long way from a uniformly fatal condition to long-term survivors with near normal quality of life. The operative approach has shifted toward a minimally invasive approach at tertiary centers. This has progressed well for the last 24 years since its beginning. Elucidating historical perspectives of an operation helps surgeons to understand and innovate with the procedure. This chapter has presented a concise account of 300 years of history for surgery of esophageal atresia. This will help to generate further interest in the nuances of thoracoscopic repair of esophageal atresia presented in this book.

Acknowledgements The author thanks Prof Raveenthiran Venkatachalam for reviewing the manuscript and providing valuable comments.

References

1. Schlee D, Teilen TM, Fiegel H, Hutter M, Rolle U. Outcome of esophageal atresia: inborn versus outborn patients. Dis Esophagus. 2022;35(8):doac001.
2. Bell JC, Baynam G, Bergman JEH, Bermejo-Sanchez E, Botto LD, Canfield MA, et al. Survival of infants born with esophageal atresia among 24 international birth defects surveillance programs. Birth Defects Res. 2021;113(12):945–57.
3. Schmedding A, Wittekindt B, Schloesser R, Hutter M, Rolle U. Outcome of esophageal atresia in Germany. Dis Esophagus. 2021;34(4):doaa093.
4. Durfton W. A narrative of a monstrous birth in Plymouth together with the anatomical observations, taken there upon by William Durston Doctor in Physik, and communicated to Dr. Tim Clerk. Philos Trans Lond. 1670;5:2096.
5. Gibson T. The anatomy of humane bodies epitomized. 5th ed. London: Awnsham and Churchill; 1697.
6. Hill TP. Congenital malformation. Boston Med Surg J. 1839;21(20):320.
7. Hirschsprung H. Den medfedte Tillukning af Spiserpret samt Bidrag til Kundskabom den Medfodte Tyndtarmstillukning. Afhandling for den medicinske Doktorgrad, Kjebenhavn, 1861, Abstract in Medico-Chirurgieal Review. 1862;30: 437–442.
8. Mackenzie M. Malformations of the Oesophagus, Arch. Laryngology. 1880;301–315.
9. Brennemann J. Congenital atresia of the esophagus, with report of three cases. Am J Dis Child. 1913;V(2):143–50.
10. Richter H. Congenital atresia of the oesophagus: an operation designed for its cure. Surg Gynecol Obstet. 1913;17:397–402.
11. Gage M, Ochsner A. The surgical treatment of congenital tracheo-esophageal fistula in the new-born. Ann Surg. 1936;103(5):725–37.
12. Lanman TH. Congenital atresia of the esophagus: a study of thirty-two cases. Arch Surg. 1940;41(5):1060–83.
13. Ladd WE. The surgical treatment of esophageal atresia and tracheoesophageal fistulas. N Engl J Med. 1944;230(21):625–37.
14. Langston HT. The first successful total repair of congenital atresia of the esophagus with tracheoesophageal fistula. Ann Thorac Surg. 1984;38(1):72–4.
15. Nakayama DK. The history of surgery for esophageal atresia. J Pediatr Surg. 2020;55(7):1414–9.
16. Waterston DJ, Carter RE, Aberdeen E. Oesophageal atresia: tracheo-oesophageal fistula. A study of survival in 218 infants. Lancet. 1962;1(7234):819–22.
17. Ladd WE, Swenson O. Esophageal atresia and tracheo-esophageal fistula. Ann Surg. 1947;125(1):23–40.
18. Manning PB, Morgan RA, Coran AG, Wesley JR, Polley TZJ, Behrendt DM, et al. Fifty years' experience with esophageal atresia and tracheoesophageal fistula: beginning with Cameron Haight's first operation in 1935. Ann Surg. 1986;204(4):446–53.
19. Lobe TE, Rothenberg S, Waldschmidt J, Stroedter L. Thoracoscopic repair of esophageal atresia in an infant: a surgical first. Pediatr Endosurg Innov Tech. 1999;3(3):141–8.
20. Rothenberg S. Thoracoscopic repair of a tracheoesophageal fistula in neonate. Pediatr Endosurg Innov Tech. 2000;4:150–6.
21. Holcomb GW III, Rothenberg SS, Bax KM, Martinez-Ferro M, Albanese CT, Ostlie DJ, et al. Thoracoscopic repair of esophageal atresia and tracheoesophageal fistula: a multi-institutional analysis. Ann Surg. 2005;242(3):422.

Anatomy of Neonatal Chest and Mediastinum in Relation to Thoracoscopy and Esophageal Atresia

2

Contents

Learning Objectives

1. General anatomical aspects of neonatal rib cage
2. Surface anatomy of chest in right lateral position
3. Clinical anatomy of right hemithorax from the eyes of a telescope

---

Supplementary Information The online version contains supplementary material available at https://doi.org/10.1007/978-981-97-5695-7_2.

R. P. Kanojia, *Thoracoscopic Repair of Esophageal Atresia*,
https://doi.org/10.1007/978-981-97-5695-7_2

2.1 Introduction

From a surgeon's perspective, the neonatal rib cage and mediastinum are complex body cavities. In the past, the surgical repair of esophageal atresia eluded the surgeons because the area was too difficult to approach and understand the miniature tissues of the neonate. It was in the early 1900, when Richter [1] first approached mediastinum via posterior thoracotomy in an attempt to ligate trachea-esophageal fistula. He was on the right track, but unfortunately, none of his patients survived due to a lack of anesthesia and intensive care support. In the current era, thoracotomy is a standard practice for the repair of esophageal atresia. Opening the thorax and directly visualizing the anatomical structures greatly enhance the procedure's efficiency. To do the same procedure by minimal access, the surgeon must first visualize the surface and internal anatomy. This is to place the ports for repair correctly. Any experienced minimal-access surgeon will visualize the surface anatomy and see through all the invisible structures. To achieve this level of understanding, one must thoroughly know the regional anatomy.

There are ample literature descriptions available that will describe the musculoskeletal anatomy of the chest. Further details in this regard are out of the scope of this chapter. The literature lacks information on applied anatomy, specifically for a neonate. In the current scope of this chapter, we will describe the applied regional anatomy, explicitly relating to thoracoscopy for esophageal atresia.

2.2 Neonatal Rib Cage

General geometry: The rib cage of a newborn is a cylindrical structure with the anterior-posterior and transverse diameters being nearly the same. The size proportion, compared to the abdomen, is nearly 1:1 [2]. The diaphragm between the abdominal and chest cavity is not a flat partition and is more arched in newborns than in infants, toddlers, and adolescents. The right diaphragm is higher because of the relatively large liver. The Left diaphragm can also reach a higher level due to a large stomach bubble due to tracheoesophageal fistula. This is a crucial point to consider when the surgeon is estimating the anatomic space available to him inside the thorax.

2.2.1 Intercostal Space

The intercostal space in neonates is narrow, and the groove carrying the neurovascular bundle is shallow, exposing them to trauma while placing the ports. This is why, while inserting the ports, the sharp instrument entering the intercostal space should have a starting point closer to the upper border of the lower rib of that space. The intercostal space is pierced multiple times during thoracoscopy. Three times for the three ports and then once if a chest wall hitch stitch is taken where the needle enters from outside loops around the lower pouch and exits from the same intercostal space. Figure 2.1 shows the preferred entry point to avoid damage to the neurovascular bundle. The intercostal space width along its length is not uniform from posterior to anterior. The space is narrowest at the posterior end, near the costovertebral joint. It becomes wider as we move toward the lateral chest wall and then again becomes narrow toward the midline (Fig. 2.2). Similarly the higher the intercostal space, the narrower is the width and is maximum in the middle of the chest, somewhere between the sixth and seventh ribs. This is important anatomically from the perspective of placing ports and chest tubes in the neonatal chest.

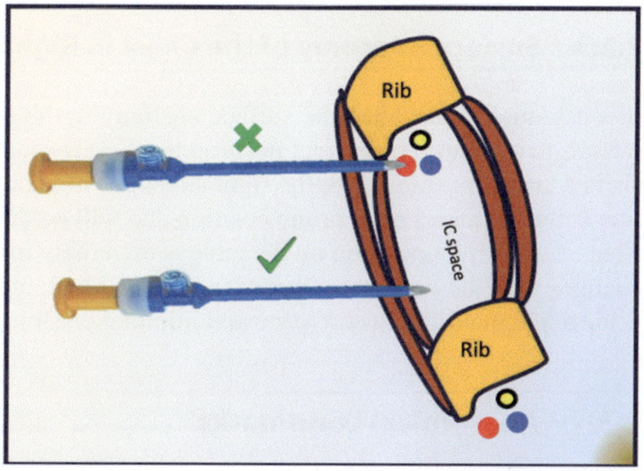

Fig. 2.1 Schematic representation of intercostal space showing the relative position of neurovascular bundle and preferred point of trocar entry

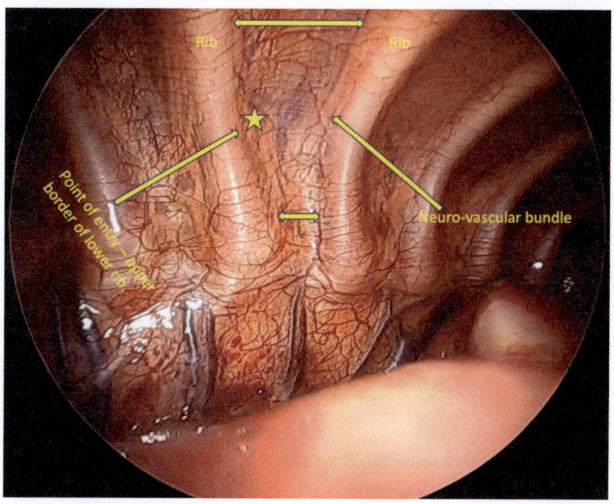

Fig. 2.2 Inside view of intercostal space showing position of neurovascular bundle and the relative breadth of the space in relation to costovertebral junction. * is the preferred point of entry of trocar preventing injury to neurovascular bundle

2.2.2 Neonatal Rib

The neonatal rib is a very flexible and arching bone. The rib can be pressed along its curvature and can bear the shearing stress of a fulcrum point for the thoracoscopy port. The rib of a neonate is virtually unbreakable unless extreme crushing forces are applied. When a port is placed between two ribs, the telescope acts as a lever, and the lower rib will offer some resistance to the vertical movement of the scope. The neonatal rib, being flexible, will bend easily in the apex of its arch and is not a problem for the camera-holding person. This contrasts with the rib in a grown-up child or adult where the rib is relatively stiff and will give shearing forces to the lower and upper rib and to the shaft of the telescope.

2.2.3 Surface Anatomy of the Chest in Right Lateral Position

It is essential to visualize the surface anatomy in the surgical position the surgeon intends to operate. The correct position for thoracoscopic repair of esophageal atresia is a lateral position with the right side up. The more accurate term for the position is three-quarter right prone position and will be described in more detail under Chap. 5. A correct position on the table is extremely important. The margin of error changes with the port placement ergonomics. The target is to space out the ports to achieve the maximum workspace and minimal clashing of instruments.

2.3 Anatomical Landmarks

There are four most important anatomical landmarks (Fig. 2.3). The inferior angle of the scapula and the right areola are the two visible landmarks. The other two landmarks are the subcostal border and the sixth intercostal space in the midaxillary line.

2.3.1 Inferior Angle of Scapula

This is a floating landmark which will change its position with the movement of the right hand, and therefore it is vital to fix the right arm. The arm is flexed at the shoulder and elbow joint to rest over the right ear. Once the arm is fixed in this position, the inferior angle of the scapula will be a fixed point and just below and posterior will be the TE fistula and the area where maximum dissection will be carried out.

2.3.2 Right Areola

This is the medial landmark and should be always visible in a draped patient. The right-hand port will be placed in relation to this landmark and the intercostal space is decided from inside.

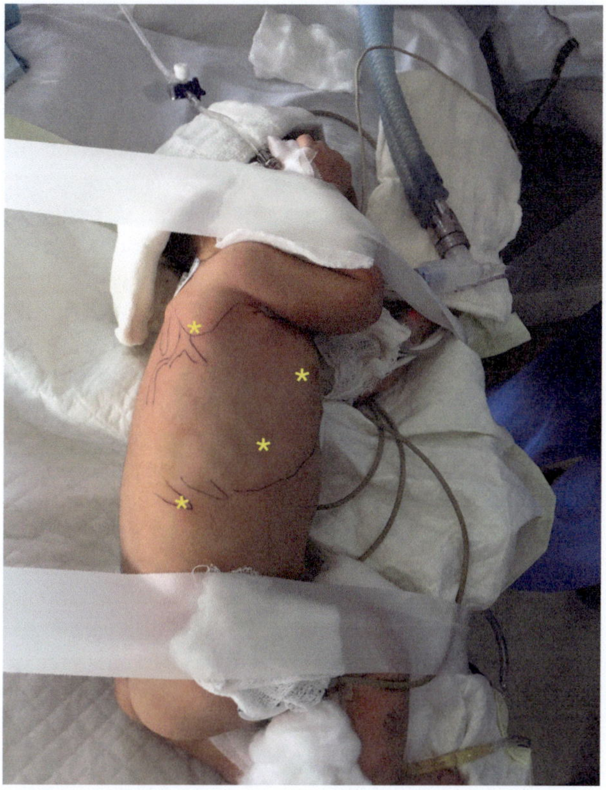

Fig. 2.3 Surface anatomy in a neonate positioned for TREAT. Important landmarks and the presumed location of upper pouch and fistula are drawn

2.3.3 The Costal Margin

This is the lower limit of your working area and the tip of the 11th and 12th ribs should be marked. This will help the surgeon to get to the lowest possible intercostal space for left-hand port placement. The nuances of this are described in the relevant sections. It's important to understand that the diaphragm is not present at this level and is present higher up as an arched structure with dome toward the thorax.

2.3.4 The Sixth Intercostal Space Midaxillary Line

This is a presumptive landmark once we have marked the above-described three points as shown in the clinical picture. This is the entry point for the first optical port which is done by open method. There is no strict rule for the intercostal space number, and one can go a space above or below depending on the geometrical perceptions at the time of planning of ports after draping with the basic idea of spacing out and achieving maximum working distance. The arching diaphragm is the most important consideration for this. If placed too low, the port may enter the subdiaphragmatic space and injure the fragile liver.

2.4 Clinical Anatomy of the Right Hemithorax (as Viewed by Telescope)

The right hemithorax is a potential space which is created by pneumatic inflation between parietal and visceral pleura and reflecting the lung away from vertebrae. The view obtained at open thoracotomy is markedly different from what is seen on thoracoscopy, the latter being superior and virtually every anatomic structure ranging from a large vascular structure as superior vena cava to smallest as the thoracic sympathetic ganglia chain. The figure displays the anatomy of the right hemithorax in a patient with esophageal atresia. The geometric shape of this area is shaped like a cone with the tip of the cone cutoff (Fig. 2.4), being narrow in the upper part. For the sake of description, it is important to understand what is medial and what is lateral. It becomes confusing for the novice while reading descriptions because most of the time, the descriptions are made as per standard position of supine patient. This is not the same for thoracoscopic view as the child is semi-prone. So, the author proposes a standard quadrant-based description as seen on the circular field of view on screen.

The circle of the field of view on screen can be divided into the upper and lower hemicircles through a diameter line which will run along the horizontal part of the azygos vein (Fig. 2.5). Anything toward the vertebrae is posterior and toward lung hilum is medial. Anything above the horizontal part of azygos vein is superior and below is inferior. The upper half of the hemicircle is the thoracic inlet, which is a busy area with major vessels as subclavian vein and artery with its branches and the superior vena cava. This also has the upper pouch covered by the endothoracic fascia. This is a tapering area, and the space is extremely limited. Any kind of suturing

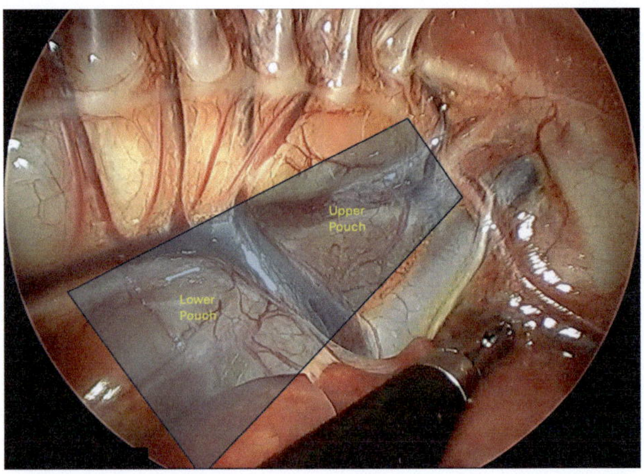

Fig. 2.4 Right thoracoscopy view emphasizing the geometric shape of the mediastinum like a cone with its tip cutoff

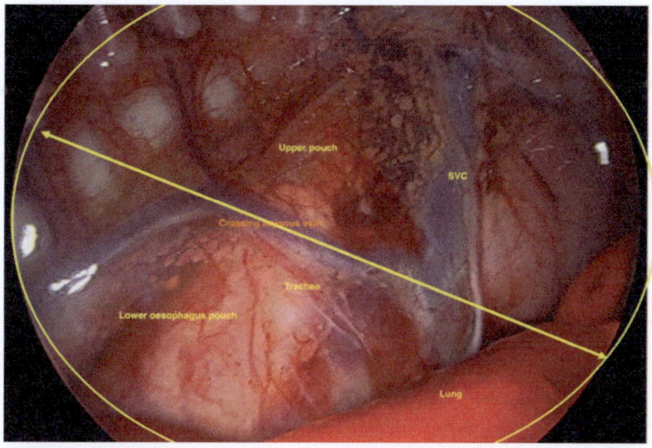

Fig. 2.5 Circle of field of view during right thoracoscopy. The diameter line passing through azygos vein

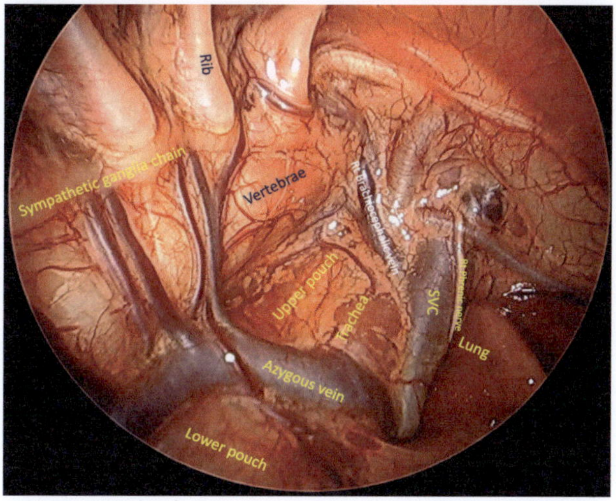

Fig. 2.6 Initial anatomy seen during TREAT

in this area is difficult as the space needed to rotate the needle is limited. The lower half of the circle of field of view will have the lower esophageal pouch which will be seen distending with ventilation. The aorta if anatomically normal will be seen alongside the lower esophageal pouch and is seen pulsating. The vagus nerve will be seen lying medial to the esophagus. In a most favorable scenario where the upper pouch is at T4, the surgeon will be doing anastomosis at the level of the diameter line which will permit maximum freedom of movement. Figure 2.6 shows the anatomy seen at the beginning of TREAT.

Another important point of applied anatomy is the requirement of closure of rib space after port removal. After port removal the intercostal space does not collapse on its own and will be like a punched-out hole in the chest wall. If this is not properly closed, it can cause life-threatening complications like pneumothorax or subcutaneous emphysema.

2.5 Conclusion

To conclude the neonatal chest and mediastinum are an anatomically crowded zones, and good ergonomics cannot be achieved unless a clear understanding of surface and internal anatomy is known. Knowing the anatomy eliminates the size scare for the operating surgeon in a neonate and gives confidence.

References

1. Richter HM. Congenital atresia of the oesophagus: an operation designed for its cure. Surg Gynecol Obstet. 1913;17:397–402.
2. Schwend RM, Schmidt JA, Reigrut JL, Blakemore LC, Akbarnia BA. Patterns of rib growth in the human child. Spine Deform. 2015;3(4):297–302.

Suggested Reading

Kanojia R. Thoracoscopic repair of esophageal atresia (unedited video). You Tube; 2020. https://youtu.be/CpZrisvHKWc?si=7kkufVt0O6YEx_h7.

Case Selection, Basic Instrumentation, and Operation Theatre Layout for TREAT

3

Contents

Learning Objectives

1. How to choose the eligible patient for TREAT
2. Contraindications for the procedure
3. Instrument requirements
4. Operation theatre layout for the hardware around the patient

3.1 Introduction

Case selection for TREAT is subjective and depends on the stage of your learning curve. It is assumed that a surgeon who is attempting TREAT is already at an advanced skill level where he understands the equipment and ergonomics and is competent for intracorporeal suturing. Thoracoscopic repair of esophageal atresia lies at the apex of the learning pyramid in minimal-access surgery. The beginner surgeon must look for the best-case scenario while attempting his early cases and try to minimize conversion and time taken for the procedure. This helps to gain

R. P. Kanojia, *Thoracoscopic Repair of Esophageal Atresia*, https://doi.org/10.1007/978-981-97-5695-7_3

confidence with the anesthesia and the rest of the operation team. Often, with first few cases at any center, the entire team is learning including the camera person, the anesthetist, and the scrub team. The dynamics of a team where all the members are novice is different from an experienced members' team. There can be mistakes and forced errors which need to be avoided. There are for essential components for this team which can be compared to the four driving wheels of a car. The surgeon and the anesthetist are the two front wheels, and the camera assistant and the scrub nurse are the two rear wheels. If either one of the components is not working efficiently, it will slow down the entire car, and it may not reach its final destination. This chapter aims to describe the most crucial components of TREAT even before you begin. It will describe how to select the eligible case and set up for small-space ergonomics. Another section also covers on the basic minimum instruments required for completing the procedure.

3.2 Case Selection

The best-case scenario for TREAT is a patient who fulfills the below criteria [1]:

1. Good weight (2.5 kg and above)
2. Isolated Ty IIIb esophageal atresia with fistula with no cardiac anomaly
3. Upper pouch at T3–T4 as seen on chest X-ray
4. Good lung condition with no features of pneumonia
5. Hemodynamically stable neonate without inotropes and no features of sepsis

Figure 3.1 shows a case selected on X-ray findings with upper pouch at T4, good lungs, and normal heart.

Once the above five conditions are met, the patient can be posted after optimization. Almost all patients will require postoperative ventilation after surgery; hence a ventilator bed should be available for the patient.

With increasing cases and a good learning curve, some of these five criteria can be made flexible, and depending on the confidence of the team, smaller and more complex cases can be done thoracoscopically. Of these weight and atresia gap are the two most common variables which become flexible. In authors' experience weight as low as 1300 g and gap as long as >2.5 cm have been successfully attempted. Dingmann et al. [2] listed 2000 g as the minimum weight criteria in their series.

There are some factors which preclude the procedure and are not controllable. Severe cardiac anomaly with unstable patient is once such contraindication for attempting TREAT. This is discussed in more detail in the Controversies chapter (Chap. 13).

Patients on high-frequency ventilation and on multiple inotropes are also a time stage contraindication. Once this baby is switched to conventional ventilation and is on single inotrope, he/she can be considered for TREAT.

There are several instances when the neonate is posted for TREAT. At the start when he is positioned on table for surgery, the saturation drops. It is always

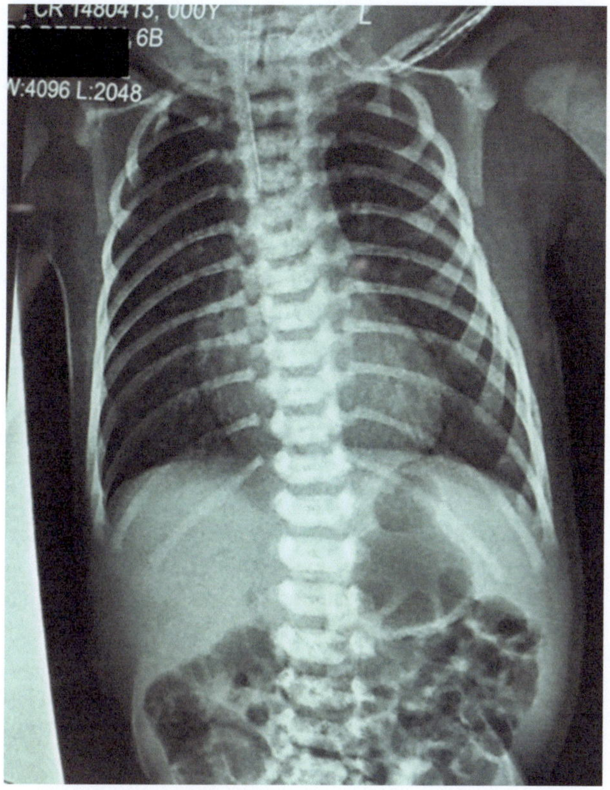

Fig. 3.1 Chest X-ray showing features of most suitable patient during case selection with upper pouch at T4, good lungs, and normal heart shadow

important to overserve the saturation for some time after final positioning is done. There may be an initial drop, but with proper ventilation, saturation picks up, and the surgeon can proceed. In some situations where the baby is not properly optimized, the fluctuations in the saturation are very wide and do not stabilize even after a period of ventilation. This commonly happens when the right lung is affected by aspiration pneumonia and the good left lung is dependent which is not ventilated/perfused to full capacity. The patient in such cases needs to be made supine again and watched for stability. A collective decision with the anesthetist is then taken for the surgical plan. This may be a candidate for open surgery.

The other reasons observed by the author for baby not maintaining after positioning are the following:

(a) Tube displacement after positioning
(b) Right bronchial intubation
(c) Ventilation into the fistula causing abdominal distention

The techniques on how to avoid these are described in the relevant section of this book (Chap. 4).

3.3 Instrumentation and Hardware

3.3.1 Ports

The minimal-access instruments are no different from what you may have been using for other neonatal procedures. Starting with the choice of ports an ideal port is one which is lightweight and has a small hub. Metal ports are heavy and not the ideal choice as the flap or the ball valve with these ports offers considerable resistance and there is a good chance of port dislodgment with the exchange of instruments. The 5 and 3 mm disposable ports if available are a good choice as they are lightweight, and the soft rubber flap valve permits easy needle movements through it. The valveless 3 mm ports are not recommended as they constantly lose inflation once the instrument is out. Fixation of ports is very important. One must note that the port must accurately be in position and because of the small working distance, the tip of the port cannot be too much inside the chest. Neither can it be too shallow in the chest. Figure 3.2 is showing three port positions: too much in, too less in, and correct position. Position A will reduce the working distance, and position B can cause frequent dislodgement. Frequent dislodgement causes loss of pneumothorax, and the working area collapses due to lung expansion. This has a twofold problem of increasing the total duration of the procedure and increasing the overall difficulty. Both will increase the surgeon's fatigue, and there will be more chances of conversion to open. The best way is to have a rubber cuff made from a glove finger and wrapped tightly around the tip Fig. 3.3 Self retaining port made with two rubber glove cuff of the port. This can be fixed with the skin using a silk suture.

There are options for a self-retaining balloon port that fixes the port. These ports are 5.5 mm and are seemingly large for a small newborn. The authors have used a double glove cuff to imitate the balloon ports (Fig. 3.3). The tip of the port is loaded with two glove finger cuffs. The lower one is smaller than the upper one. The lower one is made to enter the chest wall and act as a retainer. This virtually fixes the port and prevents any in-and-out movement. The inside cuff is tailed with a small length

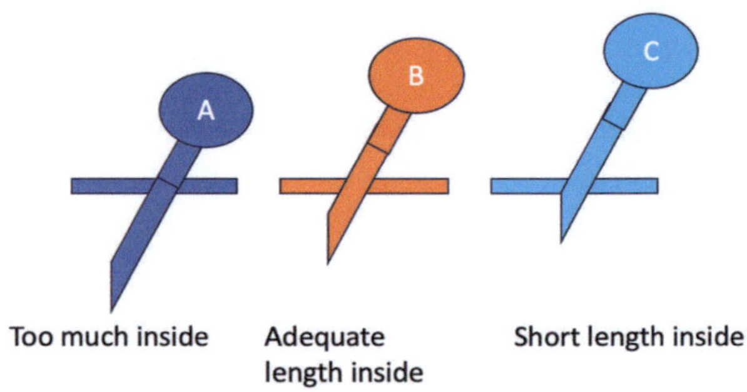

Fig. 3.2 Correct position for length of port placed inside the chest

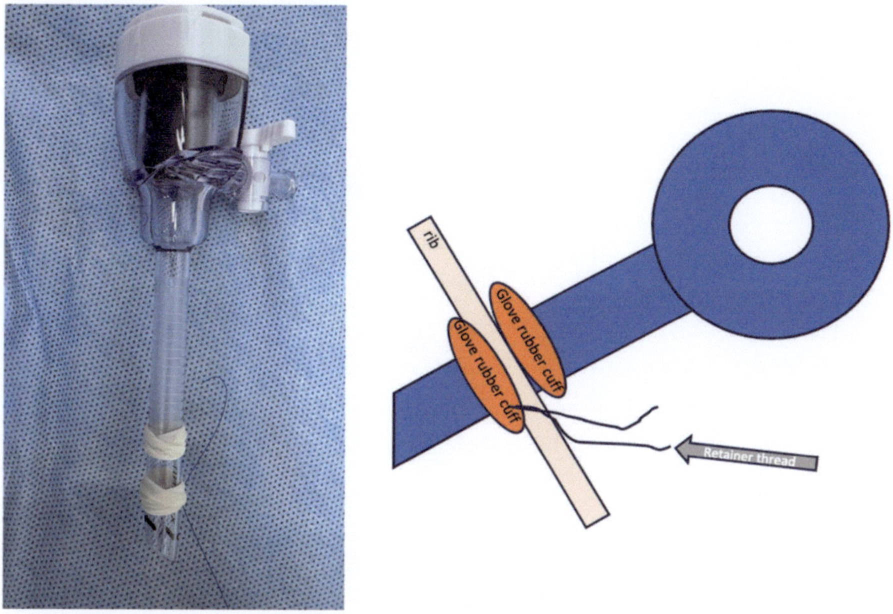

Fig. 3.3 Self-retaining port made with two rubber glove cuff

of a Prolene thread that lies outside. This is to prevent losing the inside cuff in the chest cavity.

3.3.2 Hand Instruments

Hand Instruments: basic hand instruments required are scissors (blunt tip), Maryland grasper, nontraumatic grasper, hook cautery, suction tip (trumpet suction preferable), and a curved tip needle driver. This is the basic set of instruments which should be available (Fig. 3.4). Apart from this one may require a 5 mm harmonic to tackle the azygos vein and a Hemolock clip applicator for the fistula ligation. The choice of these instruments can be 5 or 3 mm depending on the overall planning. The ideal length of these instruments is 15 cm, but the longer 25–30 cm instruments are equally good.

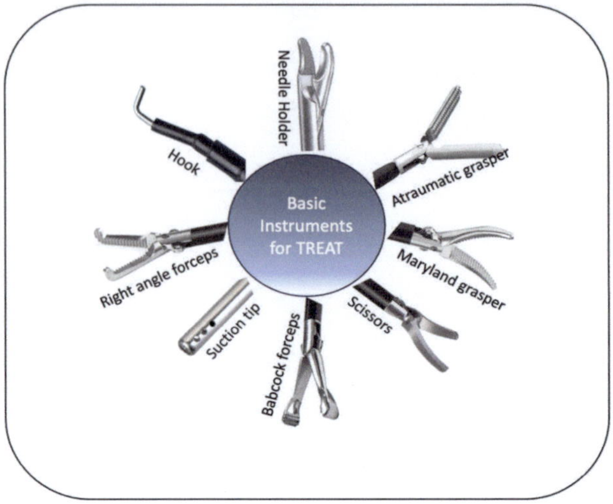

Fig. 3.4 Laparoscopic hand instruments required for procedure

3.4 Operation Theatre Layout

Planned ergonomics and operation theatre layout are extremely important to increase the efficiency of the working team. There should be no last-minute confusion on what goes where in the operating room. The best way is to make a chart or a handmade drawing on the operation theatre board explaining the layout of various equipment in the room. With the patient positioned, the surgeon will be standing on the left side of the table with the monitor in front of him. Figure 3.5 represents a diagrammatic representation of the OT layout with various components. It is always preferable to have minimum of two monitors placed at right angles. One of the monitors should be easily accessible to the anesthetic personnel so that he is able to see what's happening on the screen and synchronize with the hand movements of the surgeon. This is extremely important as the anesthetist is heavily invested in this surgical procedure, and he must sit through the procedure to maintain critical vitals.

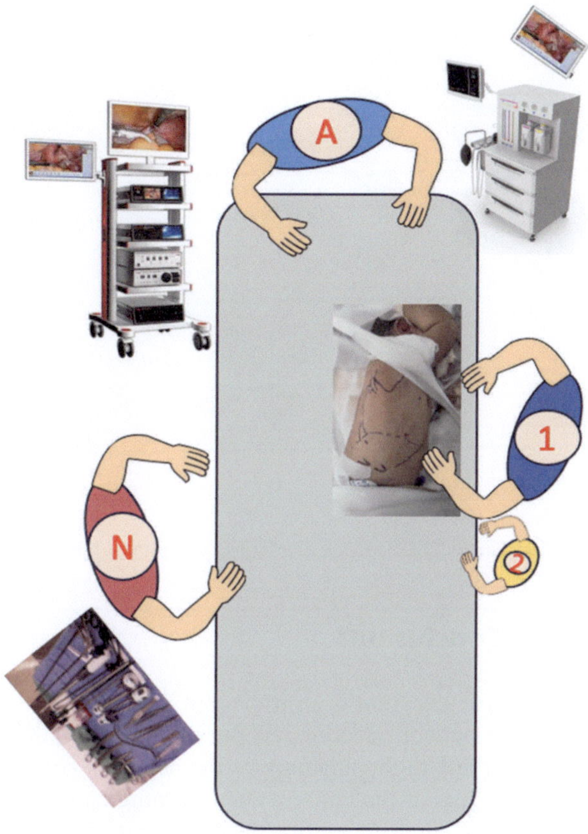

Fig. 3.5 Operation theatre layout for TREAT

3.5 The Surgeon-Camera-Organ-Picture (SCOP)

As per the general principles of laparoscopy the surgeon-camera-organ-picture should be in a straight line [3]. This is arrangement is depicted in Fig. 3.6. Maintaining this straight line will help to reduce parallax, forbid unnecessary movements, and prevent operative fatigue both for the surgeon and other team members. The hand-eye coordination will be better if this line is maintained. The monitor should be as low as possible to prevent posture fatigue.

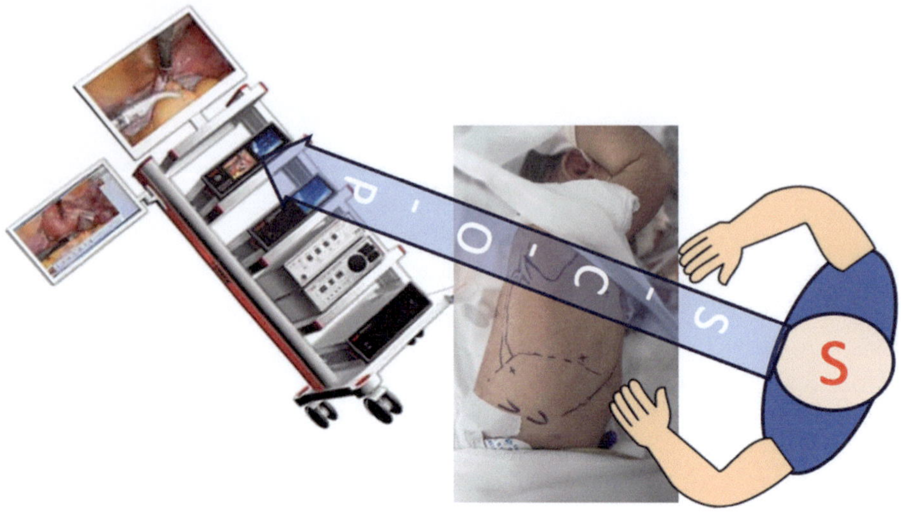

Fig. 3.6 The SCOP (Surgeon-Camera-Organ-Picture) principle for minimal-access procedures

3.6 Conclusions

Correct case selection is an important first step for a successful TREAT. With the criteria for patient selection laid out in this description, the surgeon will face fewer challenges due to the anatomy of the neonate. The adaptability for more complex cases improves as the entire team's learning curve progresses. The surgeon should be well versed in the operation theatre layout, and a pre-planned layout diagram will help to avoid confusion. The basic principles of SCOP should be followed to increase efficiency and prevent fatigue. No particular instrument is needed from what the set may already have in the laparoscopy set.

References

1. Kanojia RP, Bhardwaj N, Dwivedi D, Kumar R, Joshi S, Samujh R, et al. Thoracoscopic repair of esophageal atresia with tracheoesophageal fistula: basics of technique and its nuances. J Indian Assoc Pediatr Surg. 2016;21(3):120–4.
2. Dingemann C, Ure BM. Minimally invasive repair of esophageal atresia: an update. Eur J Pediatr Surg. 2013;23(3):198–203.
3. Madhok B, Nanayakkara K, Mahawar K. Safety considerations in laparoscopic surgery: a narrative review. World J Gastrointest Endosc. 2022;14(1):1–16.

Suggested Reading

Esposito C, Becmeur F, Steyaert H, et al. ESPES manual of pediatric minimally invasive surgery. Cham: Springer; 2019.
Parikh DH, Crabbe D, Auldist A, et al. Pediatric thoracic surgery. London: Springer; 2009.

Anesthesia and Ventilation for Thoracoscopic Esophageal Atresia Repair

4

Contents

Abbreviations

CHD	Congenital heart disease
CO_2	Carbon dioxide
CV	Closing volume
EA	Esophageal atresia
ECG	Electrocardiography
$ETCO_2$	End-tidal carbon dioxide
ETT	Endotracheal tube
FC	Fogarty catheter
FIO_2	Fraction of inhaled oxygen
FRC	Functional residual capacity

R. P. Kanojia, *Thoracoscopic Repair of Esophageal Atresia*,
https://doi.org/10.1007/978-981-97-5695-7_4

GA	General anesthesia
HFO	High-frequency oscillation
HPV	Hypoxic pulmonary vasoconstriction
IV	Intravenous
LA	Local anesthetic
LDP	Lateral decubitus position
MAC	Minimum anesthetic concentration
NDMR	Non-depolarizing muscle relaxant
NIBP	Noninvasive blood pressure
OLV	One-lung ventilation
PA	Pulmonary artery
$PaCO_2$	Arterial carbon dioxide
PCV	Pressure-controlled ventilation
PO	Postoperative
PPHN	Pulmonary hypertension of the newborn
PPV	Positive pressure ventilation
PVR	Pulmonary vascular resistance
RDS	Respiratory distress syndrome
SpO_2	Oxygen saturation
SVR	Systemic vascular resistance
TEF	Tracheoesophageal fistula
TIVA	Total intravenous anesthesia
TPN	Total parenteral nutrition
TREAT	Thoracoscopic repair of esophageal atresia
TV	Tidal volume
V/Q	Ventilation perfusion ratio

4.1 Introduction

Thoracic surgery in a neonate is performed for several surgical pathologies (tracheoesophageal fistula, congenital diaphragmatic hernia, anterior mediastinal tumors, congenital cystic adenoid malformation, etc.). These neonates may have concomitant syndromes or anomalies like congenital heart disease (CHD) which may impact anesthesia management as well as the outcome. Tracheoesophageal fistula (TEF) with/without esophageal atresia (EA) is a congenital anomaly with an incidence of 1:2500–3000 live births [1]. Various types of TEF have been described (Gross and Vogt classification systems), out of which EA combined with a distal fistula (C/IIIB) is the commonest [2]. The surgical repair of EA-TEF is usually performed via a right thoracotomy. Thoracoscopic approach to TEF repair is now gaining popularity as this technique is beneficial in terms of decreased surgical trauma, pain, and earlier recovery, although providing safe anesthesia to these babies is challenging [3]. An in-depth understanding of the basic principles of neonatal and thoracic anesthesia as well as the effects of carbon dioxide insufflation during thoracoscopy will help the anesthesiologist in planning an anesthesia technique which ensures a safe outcome.

This chapter aims to give an insight into the normal respiratory physiology of a neonate and the impact of thoracoscopic procedures as well as the presence of coexisting diseases on the anesthesia management. It will also discuss the preoperative optimization of the neonate, followed by techniques for securing the airway, the need for one-lung ventilation, the mechanical ventilation techniques, and postoperative problems encountered by a neonate presenting for thoracoscopic repair of TEF.

4.2 Thoracoscopic Procedures: Risk Factors

Neonates are at a higher risk of developing intraoperative hypoxia and hypercarbia during the conduct of thoracoscopic surgery. Normal respiratory physiology, anesthesia, lateral decubitus position for surgery, and carbon dioxide (CO_2) insufflation into the chest cavity are the factors which contribute to this.

4.2.1 Effect of Normal Respiratory Physiology and Anesthesia

Newborn infants, especially if born premature, have alveoli which are larger and few in number. Until the first year of life, there is absence of collateral connections between the alveoli (pores of Kohn and bronchoalveolar canals of Lambert), increasing the risk of atelectasis in dependent lung areas [4]. In addition, the lungs of preterm infants are surfactant-deficient, and this decreases the elastic recoil of the lung and interferes with lowering the surface tension.

The neonates have a highly compliant and deformable rib cage due to the horizontal alignment of the ribs, reducing the efficiency of the intercostal muscles. The diaphragm and the intercostal muscles contain less amount of Type 1 muscle fibers making them more prone to fatigue [5]. The functional residual capacity (FRC) determined by the static balance between the outward and inward recoil pressure of the chest wall and lungs, respectively, is lower in neonates than in older subjects. Due to the poor elastic properties of the lungs, small amount of collagen and less elastin to collagen ratio, lung stiffness, and recoil are affected. Because of these factors, the closing volume (CV) is greater than their FRC, and during normal tidal ventilation, there is an increased likelihood of airway closure. A neonate therefore has an increased likelihood of developing lung collapse, increased work of breathing, and diaphragmatic fatigue. Because of the above reasons, a neonate must be maintained on controlled ventilation rather than spontaneous ventilation during and after anesthesia. All the above factors contribute to poor lung compliance, reduced lung volume, widespread atelectasis, low FRC, high CV, ventilation-perfusion mismatch, and hypoxia in neonates [4]. Due to the developmental differences in respiratory physiology, general anesthesia (GA) in neonates significantly increases the chances of ventilation and perfusion (V/Q) mismatch and the risk of atelectasis. Also, there is an impaired ventilatory response to hypoxia and hypercarbia, and the anesthetic drugs further depress the respiratory control to both hypoxia and hypercarbia [6].

4.2.2 Effect of Lateral Decubitus Position

TEF surgery is done in the right lateral decubitus position (LDP), and compression of the lower dependent lung may lead to atelectasis. Neuromuscular blocking agents and mechanical ventilation during GA cause a decrease in FRC of both lungs leading to V/Q mismatch. Surgical retraction of the lung or use of one-lung ventilation (OLV) results in the collapse of the operative lung and the development of atelectasis. Hypoxic pulmonary vasoconstriction (HPV) normally diverts blood flow away from the under-ventilated lung, so as to minimize V/Q mismatch. This response may be decreased by inhalational anesthetic agents and other vasodilating drugs. Increased oxygen consumption at baseline produces a high risk of intraoperative hypoxia, which is further increased in the lateral position. These factors apply equally to patients of all age groups from infants to adults. However, the overall effect of the lateral decubitus position on V/Q mismatch is more pronounced in infants compared with older children and adults. In contrast to adult patients, pediatric patients have better oxygenation with the healthy lung uppermost which is not possible in thoracic surgery where the diseased lung is up [3]. This is partly due to a reduced hydrostatic pressure gradient between the two lungs and a compliant chest wall that does not support the underlying lungs.

4.2.3 Effect of Carbon Dioxide Insufflation

CO_2 is insufflated into the chest during thoracoscopic surgery to improve surgical visualization and prevent overdistension of the lung. This leads to a collapse of the affected side lung, limiting the lung excursion and decreasing the lung compliance. This compromises the lung function and contributes to hypercarbia and hypoxia.

In addition, venous return to the heart is reduced resulting in a decrease in cardiac output. This can occur due to excessive volume or pressure produced by excessive pneumothorax which displaces the intrathoracic contents. A slow release of CO_2 (1 L/min) and keeping the inflating pressure at <4–6 mmHg prevent these effects [6].

Development of acidosis owing to hypercarbia during thoracoscopy is likely to revert the neonate to transitional circulation. Hypercarbia causes failure of the pulmonary vascular resistance (PVR) to decrease with an increase in systemic vascular resistance (SVR) to shift the from fetal right-to-left flow to the neonatal left-to-right flow from the aorta into the pulmonary artery (PA). Because of this, there is significant mixing of blood through both the patent ductus arteriosus and patent foramen ovale, leading to hypoxia ("persistent fetal circulation") [7]. Because of this mixing, a large part of cardiac output is contributed by the right ventricle and the postductal saturation is lower than the pre-ductal saturation. A newborn is at risk of reverting to transitional circulation, especially in situations of prematurity, sepsis, respiratory distress syndrome (RDS), acidosis, and conditions like congenital diaphragmatic hernia (CDH) with persistent pulmonary hypertension of the newborn (PPHN) [8].

Embolism followed by cardiovascular collapse is another complication which can occur with the insufflation of CO_2 [9]. This can be due to the entry of gas into the systemic circulation either by direct injection into the vessels or via entry of gas into a vessel damaged during the procedure.

4.3 Anesthesia Management Goals

The main management goals an anesthesiologist should focus on for thoracoscopic repair of esophageal atresia (TREAT) surgery are avoidance of hypoxia, hypercarbia, and acidosis, maintenance of stable hemodynamics, and ensuring minimal interference with surgical visualization and manipulation [10]. The anesthesia technique therefore should focus on these considerations.

4.3.1 Preoperative Assessment and Optimization

Esophageal atresia repair is considered a surgical emergency and is usually done in the first week of neonatal life with a majority of them being done in the initial 2–3 days. The outcome after EA-TEF surgery is affected by several factors which may or may not be modifiable. Several factors are unmodifiable, namely, gestational age (prematurity), weight (low birth weight), and presence of congenital malformations (congenital heart disease) which all increase the risk of surgery and anesthesia. Several risk stratification indices are available for prognostication of these babies, out of which the modified Spitz criteria are most commonly utilized [11]. Based on these criteria, a <2 kg neonate with congenital heart disease has a survival rate of 27%; on the other hand, a >2 kg neonate without cardiac disease should have survival rates nearing 100% [12].

Certain factors are modifiable and can be optimized before surgery for a favorable outcome. These include identification and management of the presence of chest infection, CHD, assessment of hydration status, acid-base abnormalities, preoperative anemia, need for mechanical ventilation, etc. These can be optimized preoperatively to enable a good outcome and prepare the baby for anesthesia and surgery.

Neonates with EA-TEF are prone to recurrent aspirations and subsequent pneumonia owing to the communication between the esophagus and the respiratory system. The aspirations continue till surgical correction is done [12]. This is especially common where the EA-TEF has not been diagnosed at birth, oral feeds are not stopped, and the child presents late to the hospital. Therefore, oral feeds should be stopped immediately on diagnosis of the condition till surgery is done to prevent lung soiling. The neonate is nursed in a semi-upright position with continuous low-pressure suction of the upper pouch using the Replogle tube which reduces spillage into the lungs. Respiratory acidosis due to aspiration pneumonitis, atelectasis, and elevation of the diaphragm (gastric distension) leads to shunting, hypercarbia, and hypoxia especially if surgery is delayed. Antibiotics should be started for treatment of aspiration pneumonitis [13, 14].

Neonates with EA-TEF have an increased likelihood (30–50%) of having associated congenital anomalies as well as syndromes like VACTORL (v-vertebral; a-anal; c-cardiac; to-tracheoesophageal; r-renal; l-limb) [15]. The presence of cyanotic (tetralogy of Fallot) and acyanotic (ASD, VSD, PDA) congenital heart disease as well as presence of right aortic arch should be screened preoperatively by echocardiography. These cardiac anomalies affect the anesthesia management as well as the surgical outcome. In thoracoscopic surgeries since raised intrathoracic pressure compromises the cardiovascular function because of reduction in venous return, cardiac index, and mean arterial pressure, the presence of CHD needs special attention [15]. There is an increase in PVR due to hypercarbia and acidosis, thereby increasing right heart strain and right to left shunt. Some amount of hypercarbia may be helpful in some duct-dependent cardiac lesions, as maintaining PVR can help avoid pulmonary over-circulation. However, there is no scientific evidence of whether thoracoscopy causes more mortality or morbidity in neonates with CHD undergoing TEF surgery. Retrospective case series and a few case reports of thoracoscopic TEF repair done in children with CHD have shown no adverse outcome in this group of patients [16–18]. In the absence of robust evidence, prudence should be exerted when selecting such neonates for thoracoscopic procedures, and an experienced team of anesthesiologists and surgeons should be present for the same.

Respiratory distress due to either prematurity, aspiration of gastric contents, or cardiac pathology may require preoperative intubation and mechanical ventilation. However, positive pressure ventilation in context of distal fistula will cause the entry of gases into the stomach leading to gastric insufflation and regurgitation, thus worsening the already compromised ventilatory parameters. The use of synchronized ventilation techniques or volume-targeted modes of ventilation like pressure-regulated volume-controlled and volume-guaranteed techniques is therefore recommended [19, 20].

Neonates may present with dehydration and acid-base abnormalities, especially if presenting late to the hospital. Hydration status can be assessed clinically by vital signs like heart rate along with capillary refill time (<3 s), assessment of skin turgor, fontanelle fullness, hydration of mucosal surfaces, and measurement of adequate urine output (1–3 mL/kg/h). Levels of serum sodium and lactate provide biochemical evidence of the hydration status. An intravenous (IV) line is placed, and the child is given maintenance fluids (balanced salt solution with 1–2% dextrose) to ensure euvolemia and normoglycemia. If required, a central venous line can be inserted for the optimization of fluid status. Metabolic acidosis might occur due to severe dehydration leading to shock and the development of transitional circulation. Correction of acid-base abnormalities in the first 24–72 h of life before taking up for surgery is therefore important.

Presence of preoperative anemia is usually due to prematurity and increases the likelihood of postoperative apnea and hemodynamic perturbations [21]. The preoperative hematocrit also provides an idea regarding the hydration status as well as serves as a baseline for transfusion if required. The platelet and total leucocyte count are indicative of preexisting pneumonia and sepsis.

Arterial blood gas parameters coupled with oxygen saturation values are helpful in assessing if the baby will tolerate thoracoscopic repair and one-lung ventilation. While there are no current guidelines or cutoffs for the same, room air saturation less than 88% is usually not amenable to one-lung ventilation. Preexisting hypercarbia leading to pH derangement is also a relative contraindication for thoracoscopic repair.

4.3.2 Anesthesia and Securing of the Airway

Thoracoscopic surgery is conducted under GA using either inhalational (graded sevoflurane 1–8%) or intravenous agents (thiopentone 3 mg/kg, propofol 2–3 mg/kg, ketamine 2–3 mg/kg) for induction. Tracheoesophageal fistula is primarily an airway anomaly, and it may coexist with other airway malformations like tracheabronchomalacia, upper tracheal pouch, stenosis, and partial agenesis. The surgeons might opt for a preoperative assessment of the airway via rigid bronchoscopy to determine the exact site of the fistula, the presence of multiple fistulae, and associated airway anomalies [22]. This is usually done before endotracheal intubation under anesthesia.

Securing the airway by an endotracheal tube (ETT) is one of the crucial steps in the anesthesia management for surgery involving TEF repair. Positive pressure ventilation (PPV) during anesthesia leads to gastric distension especially in patients whose lungs have poor compliance secondary to aspiration and pneumonia. This distension leads to further respiratory embarrassment as well as increases the intra-abdominal pressure which may impede the venous return. In some neonates, a prior gastrostomy to relieve this distension may lead to a significant leak during ventilation.

There are two schools of thought whether the child should be intubated under spontaneous breathing or paralyzed with a **n**on-**d**epolarizing **m**uscle **r**elaxant (NDMR). The proponents of the technique of intubation under spontaneous breathing quote it's advantages as that spontaneous breathing creates negative intrathoracic pressure which causes air to enter the lungs rather than the abdomen via the fistula [23]. If maintaining oxygenation under anesthesia proves difficult, this technique allows the neonate to be awakened safely without desaturation. However, spontaneous breathing may lead to cough and gag and subsequently a poor/suboptimal glottic view. Also, the gas exchange will not be optimal without PPV if the child has a poorly compliant lung. It may be challenging to conduct rigid bronchoscopy and intubation without the use of muscle relaxants. Giving small boluses of propofol may be helpful in this situation.

Rapid sequence induction with intravenous agents and muscle relaxants (succinylcholine 2 mg/kg) without positive pressure ventilation can also be done. This leads to better and faster control of the airway as well as it avoids airway injury and intubation difficulty. Using a muscle relaxant for intubation produces optimal intubating conditions without coughing and straining as well as optimum surgical conditions. However, with the use of muscle relaxants, the anesthetic gases find the path of least resistance through the fistula to the stomach thereby causing stomach distension and risk of aspiration [24].

Awake intubation with direct laryngoscopy has been traditionally described, where the airway is anesthetized with local anesthetic jelly and spray [22]. Preoxygenation with 100% oxygen and para-oxygenation using nasal cannula can help to prolong safe apnea time till intubation and should be implemented during airway instrumentation.

After the ETT has passed the glottis, one can ensure effective ventilation and avoidance of gastric distension by several techniques. The most common technique involves deliberate endobronchial intubation and gradual withdrawal of the ETT till bilateral air entry is heard on auscultation of the lungs with minimal leak on auscultation over the stomach. The tube is rotated so that its bevel faces anteriorly and the posteriorly placed fistula is occluded by the tube [24]. Using a cuffed tube such that the tip lies below the fistula and the cuff occludes the fistula is another option for securing the airway, but it necessitates the need for bronchoscopy to confirm the ETT placement. The placement of a Fogarty catheter (FC) in the fistula under bronchoscopic guidance has also been described [25]. During bronchoscopy, ventilation should be paused once the scope is in the fistula. The balloon tip is then inflated to occlude the fistula. In cases of low-lying or large fistulas even if the ETT has been correctly placed, it can still migrate into the fistula, especially during positioning. Reconfirmation of the ETT position should be done if there is a sudden loss of ventilation or change in airway pressures.

After intubation, anesthesia is maintained with using an oxygen–air mixture [fraction of inspired oxygen (FIO_2) 0.5], avoiding nitrous oxide, intermittent doses of a non-depolarizing muscle relaxant like atracurium (0.25 mg/kg), fentanyl (0.5–1 μg/kg) for analgesia, and inhalational agent like sevoflurane or isoflurane (MAC 0.9–1). Maintenance of anesthesia should be with isoflurane preferably since it causes less attenuation of HPV. Maintenance fluids are administered based on Holliday-Segar formula [26]. The intrathoracic pressure should be kept between 4 and 6 mmHg as higher pressures may lead to transitional circulation.

4.3.3 Is One-Lung Ventilation Required?

During thoracoscopic procedures, a pressure of 4–5 cm H_2O exerted by the insufflated gas is generally adequate to deflate the nondependent lung and provide adequate space to the surgeon for the procedure to be accomplished. However, some surgeons may prefer one-lung ventilation (OLV) for obtaining a clear field for surgery thereby shortening the thoracoscopic time. To facilitate one-lung ventilation for thoracoscopic procedures, two types of techniques can be employed—(a) using Fogarty catheter (FC) as a right bronchial blocker and (b) endobronchial intubation of left bronchus with single lumen ETT [24, 25].

4.3.3.1 Placement of Fogarty Catheter

After muscle relaxation, Fogarty catheter is advanced through the glottis by direct laryngoscopy. After reaching the trachea, the catheter tip is flexed and rotated 90° to the right for right-sided placement and 90° to the left for left-sided placement, before advancing it into the desired main stem bronchus (Fig. 4.1). The catheter balloon is positioned in the proximal part of the main stem bronchus under fiber-optic visual guidance or via rigid bronchoscope. Blind placement may lead to trauma and is not advocated in neonates. The ETT is then placed beside the catheter into the trachea. The catheter is placed outside the ETT to avoid compromise of the cross-sectional area of the ETT which can impair ventilation (Fig. 4.2). The position of the FC is confirmed after the child is shifted to the lateral decubitus position. The advantage of this catheter is that it can be used even in neonates and infants (size 2.5–3F) with success. Potential problems include the following: (1) the catheter can get dislodged into the trachea, causing obstruction to ventilation. (2) Overdistension of the balloon can damage/rupture the airway because the catheter has a low-volume and high-pressure balloon. (3) These catheters do not have a central channel for suction or egress of gases or oxygen insufflation. Therefore, catheters with an open tip are preferred over closed-tip ones.

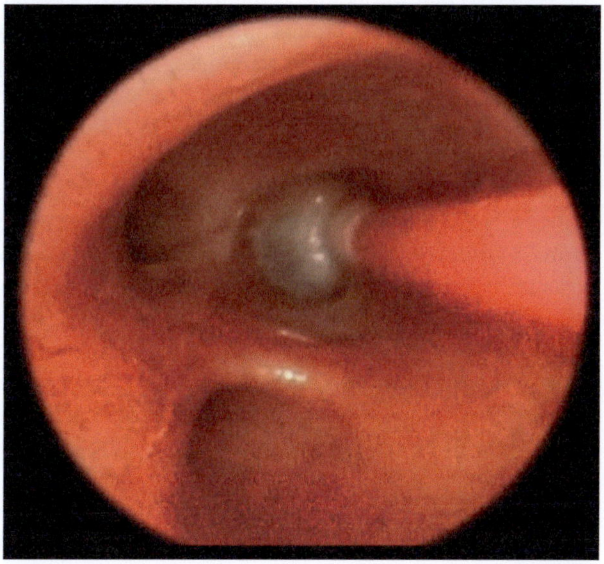

Fig. 4.1 Fogarty balloon placed with bronchoscopy assistance, occluding the right main stem bronchus

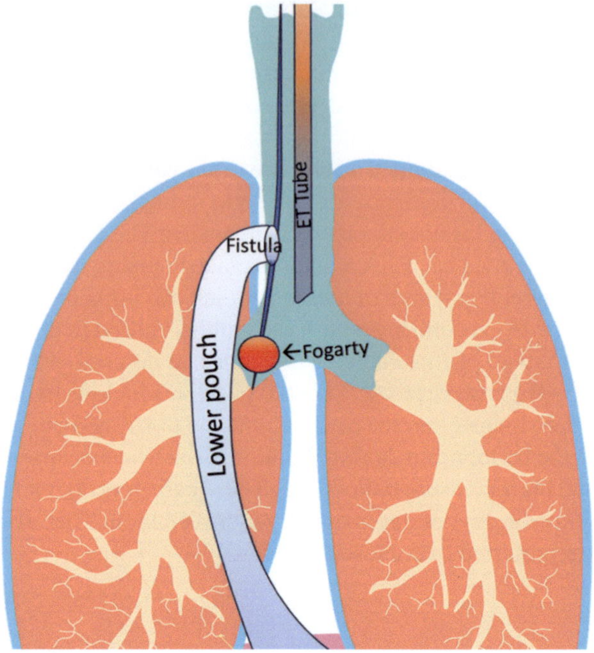

Fig. 4.2 Schematic representation of relative position of ET tube and Fogarty catheter. Note that the Fogarty comes outside the lumen of ET tube and is placed using bronchoscopic assistance

4.3.3.2 Placement of Single-Lumen ETT

For selective endobronchial intubation, a conventional uncuffed or cuffed ETT is placed intentionally into the bronchus of the nonsurgical lung. The ETT chosen for bronchial intubation needs to be smaller than the appropriate ETT by 0.5 or 1 mm. Also, the distance from the tip of the tube to the distal cuff must be shorter than the length of the bronchus to ensure that the cuff lies entirely in the bronchus. In cases of hypoxia and hypercarbia, the bronchial tube must be withdrawn for resuming two-lung ventilation; however, this can lead to an increase in airway resistance. Conversely using a larger tube for endobronchial intubation can lead to bronchial edema. Correct placement of the tube in the bronchus can be confirmed clinically or by using a fiber-optic bronchoscope. To precisely place the tip of ETT in the left lung via blind method, the technique is of hit and try. Appropriate size of ETT is taken, and a stylet is passed in the tube. With the stylet inside, the ET tube tip is bent in a way that its distal 2–3 cm makes an angle with the long axis of the remaining tube (Fig. 4.3). The tube is then passed into trachea with angulation being maintained toward the left bronchus. Once the tube has crossed the cords, keeping the angulation toward the left, the stylet is withdrawn. If the tip has successfully entered the left bronchus, then the air entry on the right side of chest will be absent with good air entry on the left side with no breath sounds in the epigastrium. This may take more than one attempt to achieve left bronchial intubation.

The advantages of this technique are that it does not require any sophisticated airway equipment and placement is easy during emergency. The disadvantages include the following: (1) it is difficult to provide an adequate seal of the bronchus

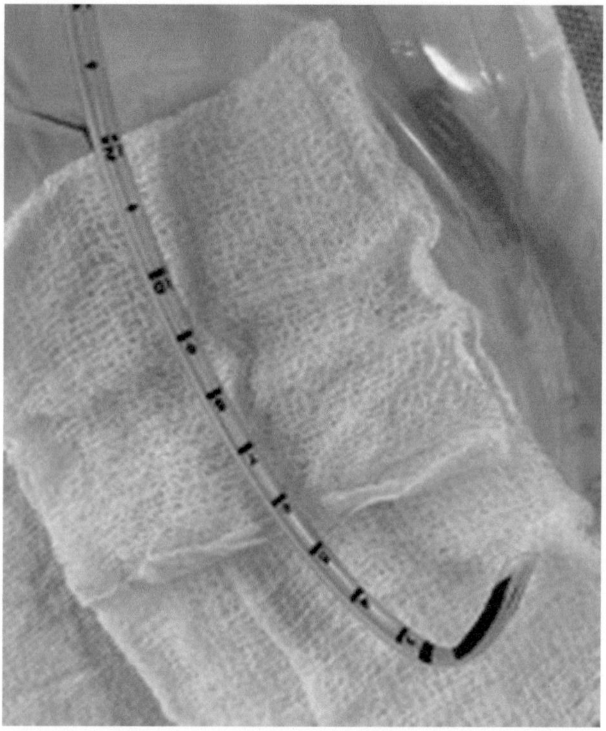

Fig. 4.3 Prepared ET tube with angulation of tip for guiding it into left main stem bronchus

preventing the operative lung from adequately collapsing and also does not prevent contamination of the healthy lung (2). Suctioning of the operated lung and providing continuous positive airway pressure cannot be done (3). Repeated attempts may lead to airway edema.

One-lung ventilation may lead to a number of problems [27]. Hypoxic pulmonary vasoconstriction (HPV) is a physiological response which reroutes blood to well-ventilated lung zones. This decreases the development of V/Q mismatch and improves oxygenation. However, HPV is obtunded during anesthesia leading to hypoxia by transpulmonary shunting of blood from right to left. A rapid CO_2 insufflation may lead to tension pneumothorax which decreases venous return and stroke volume and also produces hypotension. It can cause bradycardia, mediastinal shift, and cardiac tamponade by activating the stretch receptors and by increasing the vagal tone and can also cause prolonged collapse of the left lung lobe, and an increase in PVR that can reverse blood flow via the intracardiac shunts is likely to occur.

4.4 Ventilation Strategies

The aim of ventilation during thoracoscopic surgery is to maintain adequate oxygenation with permissible hypercarbia. Gentle ventilation of both lungs should be done as aggressive ventilation can obscure the view of the surgeon. The fraction of inhaled oxygen (FIO_2) is adjusted to target oxygen saturation (SpO_2) values of >85%. The end-tidal carbon dioxide ($ETCO_2$) values are generally inaccurate as they under read the arterial carbon dioxide ($PaCO_2$) values. Therefore, arterial blood gas sampling is desirable for accurate assessment of $PaCO_2$ and pH.

Pressure-controlled ventilation (PCV) is a ventilation strategy used mainly for neonatal thoracoscopic surgery [20]. It involves maintaining a peak airway pressure at 15–25 cm H_2O with a respiratory rate of 35–55/min, a FIO_2 of 60–80%, and an I:E ratio of 1:1–1.5. During the surgical procedure, the airway is intermittently suctioned to clear secretions. Kinking, migration of ETT, and secretions may produce high airway pressures which should be monitored by the anesthesiologist. Loss of ventilation with low airway pressures may indicate leak or slippage of the tube in a large fistula or transection of the trachea or bronchus. When the procedure is prolonged, hypercarbia leading to acidosis can set in with or without hypoxia. In such circumstances communicating with the surgical team for intermittent reinflation of the right lung by ventilation, release of CO_2, and releasing the lung retraction along with hyperventilation can facilitate CO_2 washout and improve oxygenation. High-frequency oscillation (HFO) technique of ventilation has also been described which provides a silent surgical field, maintains oxygenation, and helps in the elimination of carbon dioxide [28]. However, it needs to be coupled with total intravenous anesthesia (TIVA) as it is not an incorporated mode of ventilation in anesthesia workstations.

4.5 Monitoring

During surgery, children should be monitored by continuous five-lead electrocardiography (ECG), automated noninvasive blood pressure (NIBP), SpO_2 by pulse oximetry (preferably both pre- and postductal), capnography, exhaled tidal volume (TV), minimum anesthetic concentration (MAC), end-tidal anesthetic concentration, and temperature. Out of these, monitoring of expired TV is most important to prevent hypoventilation since children are usually ventilated with pressure control mode. During thoracic procedures especially utilizing OLV, inaccurate results may be obtained with $ETCO_2$ measurement in neonates because of alterations in dead space and shunt fractions. In this situation transcutaneous CO_2 monitoring may be an option [29]. Intravenous access should be secured in the upper limb as venous return from the lower limb may be impeded after insufflation of CO_2 in the thorax. Increase in IAP can compress the inferior vena cava and block the entry of drugs to the systemic circulation. Central venous access may be indicated if there is a possibility of the need of ionotropic support and postoperative total parenteral nutrition (TPN) and should be placed preferably on the side of the thoracoscopy. This avoids the creation of bilateral pneumothoraxes—surgical pneumothorax on the side of thoracoscopy and the unintentional pneumothorax caused by CVP line placement. Blood glucose levels should also be monitored to prevent hypoglycemia.

4.6 Postoperative Management

Postoperative pain can be managed using opioids, epidural catheters, intercostal block, local anesthetic (LA) infiltration, and paravertebral block [6]. Commonly used LAs in neonates include 0.125% bupivacaine and 0.2% ropivacaine. LA in neonates has a greater volume of distribution, which counteracts the increased potential for toxicity due to increased free, nonprotein-bound fraction. While giving continuous infusion of LA, attention should be paid to immature metabolism systems.

Some neonates get extubated on the operating table; others may need postoperative (PO) ventilation based on their prematurity, preoperative and intraoperative respiratory status, ease and duration of surgery, as well as surgical need. In some centers, elective PO ventilation for 24–48 h is mandatory in all operated TEFs. They are monitored in the neonatal intensive care unit till they are extubated.

4.7 Conclusions

Anesthesia provided to neonates undergoing thoracoscopic TEF repair needs a comprehensive understanding of the alterations of physiology caused by the procedure. Medical optimization of modifiable factors and identification of nonmodifiable risk factors for prognostication are the main components of the preoperative preparation of these babies. Securing the airway with fistula isolation, ensuring adequate oxygenation with permissive hypercarbia, and maintaining stable hemodynamics with prevention of transitional circulation form the cornerstones of intraoperative management. Lung isolation should be done in neonates with well-preserved lungs, and complications of the same should be kept in mind. Adequate analgesia in the postoperative period helps speed up the recovery of the baby. The need for postoperative mechanical ventilation should be a team decision of the operating surgeons and anesthesiologists. The body of literature on safe anesthesia practice for neonates undergoing thoracoscopic TEF repair is still growing, and more prospective trials are needed before formal guidelines for the same can be recommended.

References

1. Pinheiro PF, Simões e Silva AC, Pereira RM. Current knowledge on esophageal atresia. World J Gastroenterol. 2012;18:3662–72.
2. Spitz L. Oesophageal atresia. Orphanet J Rare Dis. 2007;2:24.

3. Tobias JD. Anaesthesia for neonatal thoracic surgery. Best Pract Res Clin Anesthesiol. 2004;18:303–20.
4. Trachsel D, Erb TO, Hammer J, von Ungern-Sternberg BS. Developmental respiratory physiology. Pediatr Anesth. 2022;32:108–17.
5. Neumann RP, von Ungern-Sternberg BS. The neonatal lung—physiology and ventilation. Pediatr Anesth. 2014;24:10–21.
6. Murray-Torres TM, Winch PD, Naguib AN, Tobias JD. Anesthesia for thoracic surgery in infants and children. Saudi J Anaesth. 2021;15:283–99.
7. Liu H, Le C, Chen J, Xu H, Yu H, Chen L, Liu H. Anesthetic management of thoracoscopic procedures in neonates: a retrospective analysis of 45 cases. Transl Pediatr. 2021;10:2035–43.
8. Zani A, Lamas-Pinheiro R, Paraboschi I, King SK, Wolinska J, Zani-RuttenstocK E, et al. Intraoperative acidosis and hypercapnia during thoracoscopic repair of congenital diaphragmatic hernia and esophageal atresia/tracheoesophageal fistula. Pediatr Anesth. 2017;27:841–8.
9. Clarke WR. The transitional circulation: physiology and anesthetic implications. J Clin Anesth. 1990;2:192–211.
10. Latham P, Dullye KK. Complications of thoracoscopy. Anesthesiol Clin North Am. 2001;19:187–200.
11. Niramis R, Tangkhabuanbut P, Anuntkosol M, Buranakitjaroen V, Tongsin A, Mahatharadol V. Clinical outcomes of esophageal atresia: comparison between the Waterston and the Spitz classifications. Ann Acad Med Singap. 2013;42:297–300.
12. Spitz L, Kiely EM, Morecroft JA, Drake DP. Oesophageal atresia: at-risk groups for the 1990s. J Pediatr Surg. 1994;29:723–5.
13. Porcaro F, Valfré L, Aufiero LR, Dall'Oglio L, De Angelis P, Villani A, et al. Respiratory problems in children with esophageal atresia and tracheoesophageal fistula. Ital J Pediatr. 2017;4:77.
14. Kovesi T. Aspiration risk and respiratory complications in patients with esophageal atresia. Front Pediatri. 2017;5:62.
15. Diaz LK, Akpek EA, Dinavahi R, Andropoulos DB. Tracheoesophageal fistula and associated congenital heart disease: implications for anesthetic management and survival. Paediatr Anaesth. 2005;15:862–9.
16. Cadaval C, Molino JA, Guillén G, Fernández SL, Hierro CL, Rodríguez MM, et al. Are low weight or cardiopathy contraindications for thoracoscopic repair of esophageal atresia with tracheoesophageal fistula? Eur J Pediatr Surg. 2024;34(4):301–5. https://doi.org/10.1055/a-2072-9754.
17. Fernandes E, Kusel A, Evans S, Houghton J, Hamill JK. Is thoracoscopic esophageal atresia repair safe in the presence of cardiac anomalies? J Pediatr Surg. 2020;55:1511–5.
18. Rice-Townsend S, Ramamoorthy C, Dutta S. Thoracoscopic repair of a type D esophageal atresia in a newborn with complex congenital heart disease. J Pediatr Surg. 2007;42:1616–9.
19. Klingenberg C, Wheeler KI, McCallion N, Morley CJ, Davis PG. Volume-targeted versus pressure-limited ventilation in neonates. Cochrane Database Syst Rev. 2017;10:CD003666.
20. Peng W, Zhu H, Shi H, Liu E. Volume-targeted ventilation is more suitable than pressure-limited ventilation for preterm infants: a systematic review and meta-analysis. Arch Dis Child Fetal Neonatal Ed. 2014;99:F158–65.
21. Welborn LG, Hannallah RS, Luban NL, Fink R, Ruttimann UE. Anemia and postoperative apnea in former preterm infants. Anesthesiology. 1991;74:1003–6.
22. Hseu A, Recko T, Jennings R, Nuss R. Upper airway anomalies in congenital tracheoesophageal fistula and esophageal atresia patients. Ann Otol Rhinol Laryngol. 2015;124:808–13.
23. Taneja B, Saxena KN. Endotracheal intubation in a neonate with esophageal atresia and trachea-esophageal fistula: pitfalls and techniques. J Neonatal Surg. 2014;3:18.
24. Broemling N, Campbell F. Anesthetic management of congenital tracheoesophageal fistula. Pediatr Anesth. 2011;21:1092–9.
25. Pepper VK, Boomer LA, Thung AK, Grischkan JM, Diefenbach KA. Routine bronchoscopy and Fogarty catheter occlusion of tracheoesophageal fistulas. J Laparoendosc Adv Surg Tech A. 2017;27:97–100.

26. Holliday MA, Segar WE. The maintenance need for water in parenteral fluid therapy. Pediatrics. 1957;19:823–32.
27. Fabila TS, Menghraj SJ. One lung ventilation strategies for infants and children undergoing video-assisted thoracoscopic surgery. Indian J Anaesth. 2013;57:339–44.
28. Zheng C, Lin Y, He Y, Shen Y, Fan J, Fang Y. Exploration of the thoracoscopic treatment of esophageal atresia under high-frequency ventilation. Front Pediatr. 2022;10:1066492.
29. Chandrakantan A, Jasiewicz R, Reinsel RA, Khmara K, Mintzer J, DeCristofaro JD, et al. Transcutaneous CO_2 versus end-tidal CO_2 in neonates and infants undergoing surgery: a prospective study. Med Dev. 2019;12:165–72.

5 Positioning Patient and Port Placement in Chest for Thoracoscopic Esophageal Atresia Repair

Contents

Learning Objectives

1. How to position neonate on operation table
2. Port planning and technique of inserting ports in neonatal chest

In thoracoscopic repair of esophageal atresia, the margin of error is small due to miniature working space for surgeon. This mandates the accuracy of the entire setup, starting from patient positioning and port placement. Once the surgeon is placed at a mechanical advantage of comfortable operating position and easy maneuverability of instruments inside the working space, he will be better able to handle the anatomical intricacies he is supposed to manage with the esophagus, trachea, and vascular structures. The rate of conversion to open is high when there is a combination of poorly positioned patient, instrument clashing, and anatomical difficulties. A good position and accurately placed ports are half the battle won. This chapter aims to eliminate the two variables of failure and conversion to open, i.e., patient positioning and port placement.

R. P. Kanojia, *Thoracoscopic Repair of Esophageal Atresia*, https://doi.org/10.1007/978-981-97-5695-7_5

5.1 Patient Positioning

Once the patient is anesthetized and handed over to the surgical team, the lead surgeon should always position the patient himself. It is not advisable for the assisting surgeons to do it as the set-up is to best suit the lead surgeon. There are several key elements to position which will be described with rationale. The initial step is to place a rigid, size 10 orogastric tube for upper pouch dissection and should be fixed in a manner that it does not interfere with the other tubes in the oral cavity and should be movable independently.

5.1.1 Position on Operation Table

The anesthetist usually has the baby at the upper end of the table for induction; hence as a first step the neonate is brought lower down in middle of the table. Thereafter lateral position is made with right side up. Making the right lateral position in the middle of the table along its breadth will make the surgeon bend his back during surgery. This is accurately depicted in Fig. 5.1. There should be enough length of the table below the baby for the scrub team to lay the cables and wires.

5.1.2 The Right Lateral Position

The conventional position for open thoracotomy repair for EA-TEF is lateral with right side up. For thoracoscopic repair the position is nearly same with some minor

Fig. 5.1 Position of neonate on operation table

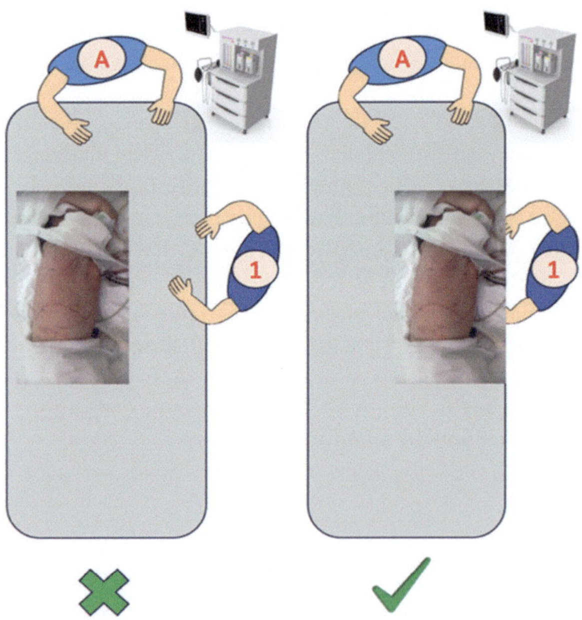

differences. The position is accurately described as **three-quarter semi-prone right lateral position.** This is achieved by first placing the patient in lateral position. Then a small soft roll is placed beneath the left chest with the aim to lift the right chest above the rest of the body. This is to follow Trendelenburg position principle. The patient is rolled slightly to make him semi-prone. The semi-prone position is stabilized with soft rolls to avoid baby becoming completely prone on his belly. The important thing to note is that there should be no rolls pressing on the abdominal wall. Too much pressure on the abdominal wall will produce ventilation problems and will also elevate the right diaphragm reducing the space in the right hemithorax. An alternative to this semi-prone position is to make the baby lateral, and then after strapping the baby, the table can be rolled with left side going up. This mimics the prone position, and the degree of prone position can be adjusted by the table tilt. The position of the right hand is important, and it should rest on the right ear with flexion at the elbow and shoulder joint. This hand position will also fix the inferior angle of scapula which forms an important landmark while planning ports (Figs. 5.2, 5.3 and 5.4).

The right leg is similarly flexed, and a soft padding is placed on the inner side of the right thigh. The left leg remains straight. This leg position will also prevent the

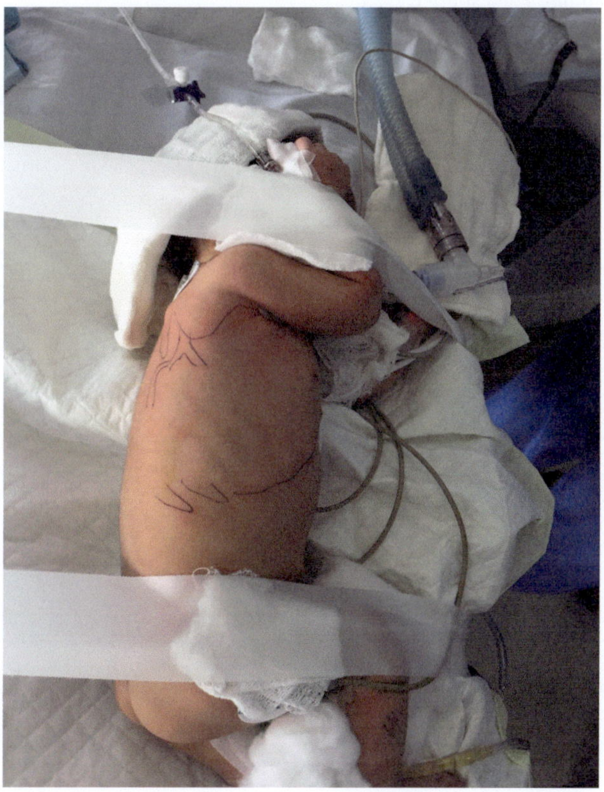

Fig. 5.2 Position of neonate. View from above

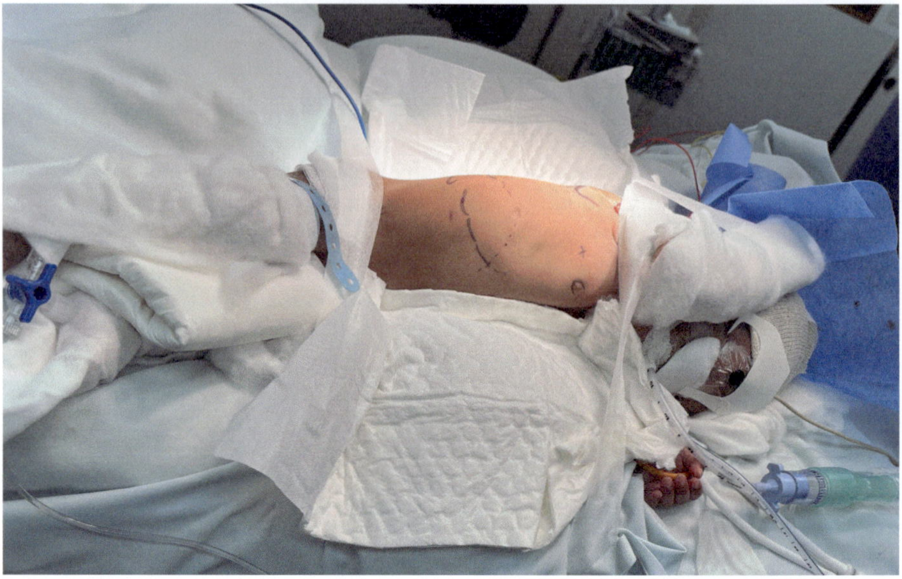

Fig. 5.3 Position of neonate. View from side. Note that the baby is closer to the left edge of table, strapped and softly padded

Fig. 5.4 Diagram to show how a three-quarter semi-prone position can be achieved by combining the roll of baby and tilt of table. Trunk of neonate is represented by the slice of CT for orientation

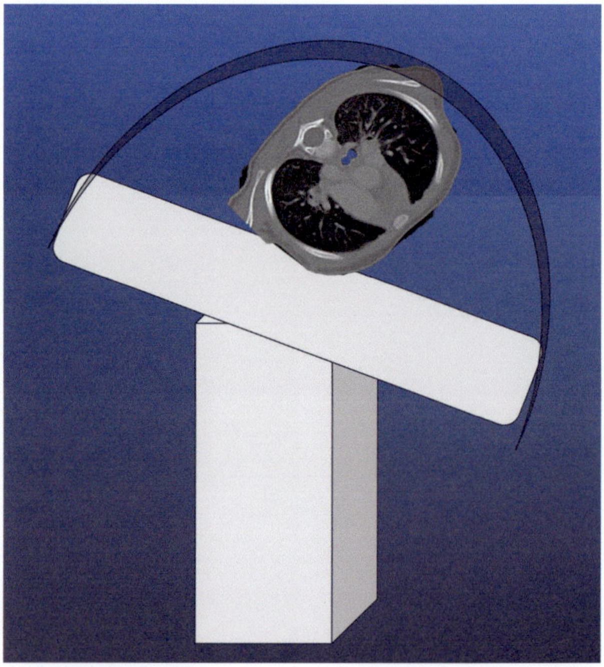

rolling of the baby on his belly. Soft padding is ensured over all pressure points. Baby is strapped by Micropore tape to fix the position on the table. The cautery plate of appropriate size can be pasted either on the thigh or the lower back. The height of the table is adjusted to the lead surgeon's height, and in general the chest of the baby should align with the elbow height. This will reduce fatigue due to shrugging of shoulders while operating.

After the final position is achieved, the baby is observed for vitals. On many occasions the baby may show a drop in saturation with rising $EtCO_2$. This happens because the good lung on the left side is dependent and compressed. In a well-prepared and optimized patient, the vitals improve with ventilation, and surgeon can proceed with the next steps. All the tubes and intravenous access line placement are now reviewed before the baby goes under the drapes. The lines should be tapped and fixed to the table to avoid dislodgement.

5.2 Port Positioning and Insertion

Once the baby is draped, the port planning is started by marking the anatomic landmarks. There are four most important landmarks for this (Fig. 5.5).

The first and most important landmark is the inferior angle of scapula (IAS). IAS is a floating point, and its position changes with the movement of right hand at shoulder joint. A fixed neutral reference position is achieved by flexing the arm at 90 deg. at shoulder joint. This point will lie in the same plane as the azygos vein, the fistula, and the site of final anastomosis. This is the space in the hemithorax which gives maximum efficiency of instruments for critical dissection. And hence the distance of the three ports should be planned in reference to this fixed IAS.

The second anatomical reference point is the right areola, and the third is the palpable subcostal margin. The tip of floating 11th and 12th ribs is marked, and the left-hand port is placed here as described in forthcoming text. The entire space bounded by the IAS, areola, right subcostal margin, and the spine posteriorly is the playground for your dissection, and the surgeon has to space out, and place his three ports following the port kite principle.

5.2.1 The Port Kite

This is a quadrilateral space formed by four reference points described above (Fig. 5.6). The point marked A is at the area where the organ of interest will be present. In this case it will be the tracheoesophageal fistula and the upper pouch. The point B is the eye or the telescope, and this is the spot for optical port. Efforts should be made to have maximum distance between A and B so that a good amount of working distance is present. This in turn increases the hand-eye coordination in the limited space. The points C and D are the entry points of the right and left working ports, and maximum efficiency of movement is achieved when the angle A is between 45° and 90°. Smaller angle will result in clashing of instruments and imbalance between the various degrees of freedom of movement (pitch yaw, roll).

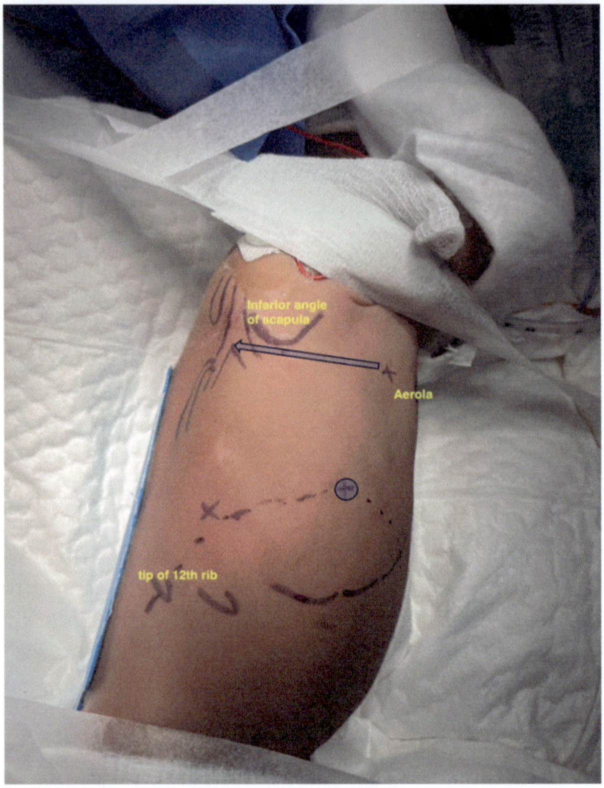

Fig. 5.5 Anatomical landmarks after positioning patient

First (optical) port is at point B which is placed by open method. The site is near the sixth or seventh intercostal space along the midaxillary line. While choosing this point, the curvature and elevation of the diaphragm are considered. The technique of insertion of port is also specific. Thereafter, an incision big enough of the size to fit a 5 mm or 3 mm port is made, and muscles are separated with artery forceps. This is very similar to the procedure of placement of chest tubes. The neonatal intercostal space is very thin, and after a gentle dissection, there is loss of resistance, which means that the tip of artery forceps is in the thoracic cavity. The opening is widened to accommodate the size of the port. The port is then gently inserted and fixed to the chest wall by sutures. The entry point of this dissection of artery forceps should be at the upper border of lower rib to avoid injury to the intercostal neurovascular bundle. More details on fixing of port are described in Chap. 3.

The correct placement of the port is confirmed by inserting the telescope and from here on the site of insertion is planned with visualization of the intercostal space from inside. For the left-hand working port, the telescope views the diaphragm, and the intercostal space just above the diaphragm insertion is seen, then light of the telescope is seen from the outside, and the site of incision is chosen. This way it will be possible to choose the lowermost intercostal space and space out for better ergonomics. If done properly this point will most likely be the seventh IC space in posterior axillary line but can vary.

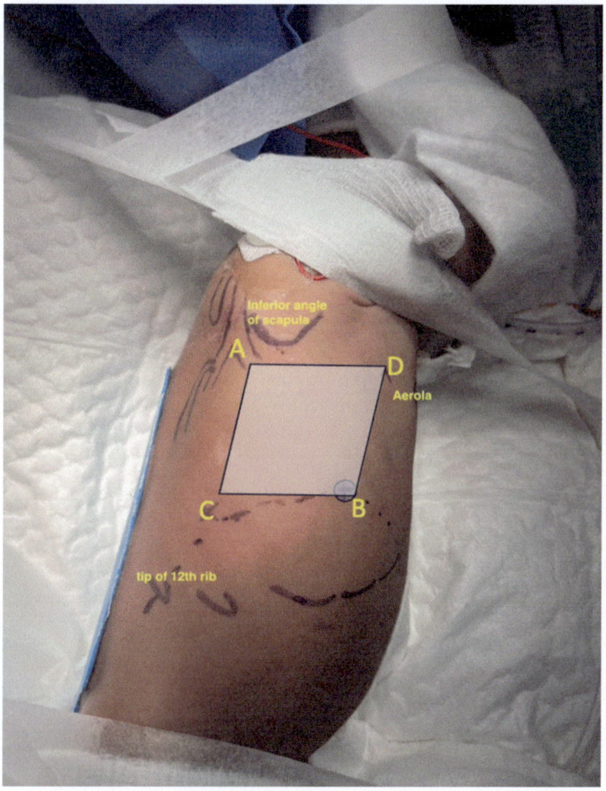

Fig. 5.6 Port kite made from joining the four anatomical reference points

Similarly, the right-hand port is placed by viewing the intercostal space from inside and will most likely be in the fourth intercostal space in anterior axillary line at the level of areola.

5.2.2 Using the Finder Needle

At times there can be discordance between the IC space seen from inside and the skin incision made on the outside. To avoid this before making the stab at the chosen skin site for port insertion, it is best to confirm the intercostal space by making a prick with a fine 26Gz needle. This will ensure that the skin incision and the point of entry of port seen from inside are the same. The finder needle is pricked at the lower border of the upper rib as a general rule.

5.2.3 Choice of Ports

The choice and size of ports depend on the surgeon and the hardware availability. Most commonly the camera port is 5 mm, and the two working ports are 3 mm. The authors have used three 5 mm ports as well as three 3 mm ports. There is not much difference in the incision size for 3 and 5 mm ports. The 5 mm ports offer the advantage of easy passage of 5/0 suture needles, 5 mm clip applicators, and vessel sealers.

Once the ports are placed, now the surgeon can proceed for the next steps of surgery.

Suggested Reading

Atlas of pediatric laparoscopy and thoracoscopy. 2008. London: Saunders/Elsevier.
Atlas of pediatric laparoscopy and thoracoscopy. 2021. Amsterdam: Elsevier Health Sciences.
Color atlas of pediatric anatomy, laparoscopy, and thoracoscopy. n.d. Berlin: Springer.
ESPES. Manual of pediatric minimally invasive surgery. Berlin: Springer; 2019.
Pediatric thoracic surgery. 2009. London: Springer.

Thoracoscopic Repair of Type C Esophageal Atresia with Tracheoesophageal Fistula with Classic Anatomy

6

Contents

Learning Objectives
To describe various steps of thoracoscopic repair of esophageal atresia in detail with classic anatomy.

Supplementary Information The online version contains supplementary material available at https://doi.org/10.1007/978-981-97-5695-7_6.

R. P. Kanojia, *Thoracoscopic Repair of Esophageal Atresia*,
https://doi.org/10.1007/978-981-97-5695-7_6

6.1 Introduction

Classic Type C or Vogt III_b esophageal atresia with tracheoesophageal fistula is the commonly encountered variant [1] (Fig. 6.1). This variant forms almost 85% of esophageal atresia occurrence. Pediatric surgeons who commonly manage esophageal atresia are always expected to be experienced with the open repair of Type C variant. With increasing practice of thoracoscopic approach, it is always advisable to start with the Type C variant at the beginning of learning curve. The anatomy is familiar constant and predictable to the operating surgeon. The only variables are the gap distance between the pouches and any vascular aberrations. The classic operation involves ligation of fistula and end-to-end esophageal anastomosis. Achieving this thoracoscopically can be technically challenging. Previous sections of this book have described various steps before the start of the actual surgical procedure, i.e., case selection, patient positioning anesthesia and port placement, etc. This chapter will elaborate, in detail, various steps of thoracoscopic repair for Type C esophageal atresia and discuss the nuances of the procedure.

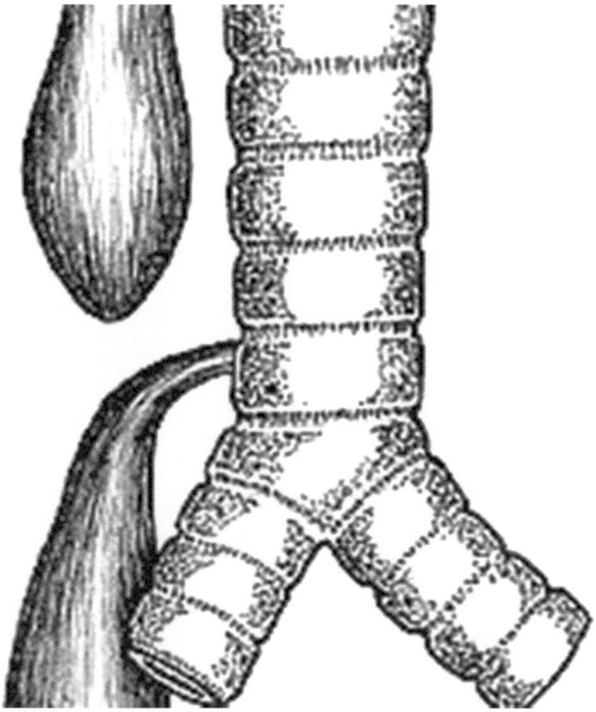

Fig. 6.1 Type C esophageal atresia with tracheoesophageal fistula. (Image credit: Wikimedia creative commons)

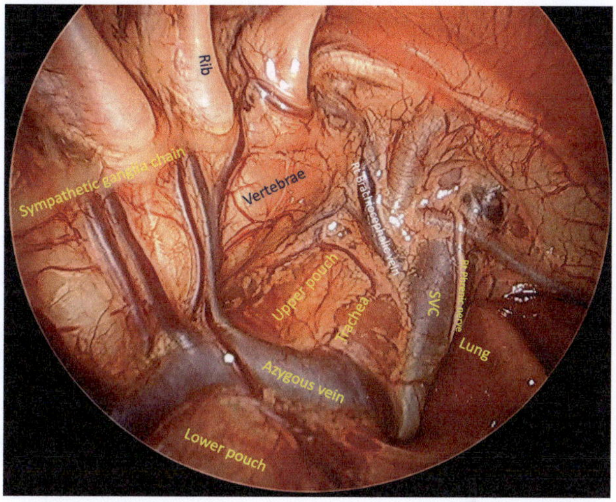

Fig. 6.2 Initial thoracoscopic view seen at the beginning. Note the general anatomy labelled with major vascular structures toward the upper half. The lung is reflected medially

6.2 Identification of Regional Anatomy

Once the operative domain is established inside the right hemithorax, right lung is made to collapse with gentle pressure by Maryland forceps. The CO_2 pressure of approximately 4–5 mm will help keep the lungs down. The right lung is gently reflected medially with an instrument to reveal the view shown in Fig. 6.2. The major landmarks identified are the azygos vein, vagus nerve, the lower pouch distending with each ventilation, and the subclavian vein in the apex of thorax. A note is taken for any aberrations in the anatomy. At this stage the feeding tube in the upper pouch is moved by the anesthetist, and the level of upper pouch is assessed. This sets the pace for the surgeon to go ahead and start with the rest of the dissection (Video 6.1).

It is important to note that during initial phase when insufflation has started and the right lung is retracted, it can result in desaturation. At the same time, touching of the vagus nerve over the lower esophagus may also cause brief desaturation episode and bradycardia. This is a normal physiological vagal response, and there is recovery with continued ventilation. There may be a requirement of momentary deflation of the chest, and the surgeon can start once the saturation and heart rate pick up. This is a kind of acclimatization response at the start of the procedure and stabilizes later with proper ventilation.

6.3 Control of Lower Pouch and Trans-fixation of Fistula

This is the first step in TREAT. It is essential that fistula should be transfixed as early as possible. This will help in better ventilation of the lungs, and patient desaturation becomes less frequent. The lower pouch usually presents itself with air distention synchronized with ventilation. There is vagus nerve overlying the lower pouch (Fig. 6.3). The endothoracic fascia is incised with hook cautery or opened with tip of Maryland dissection. The lower pouch is then gently grasped with an atraumatic bowel grasper. It is preferred to gently hitch the fistula with a looped proline suture with the chest wall (Fig. 6.4). This helps to minimize the handling of the fragile lower pouch, and the surgeon can use both hands to dissect the lower pouch up to the tracheal junction. This will also prevent air going down into stomach. The fistula is then transfixed with a nonabsorbable suture (Fig. 6.5). Once ligated the hitch is dropped without disconnecting the fistula. This is done to avoid retraction of the lower pouch. Use of clips versus suture trans-fixation is a matter of surgeon's preference. Sometimes it is done to save time in a critical and unstable patient to improve ventilation (Fig. 6.6). The authors prefer the method of suture trans-fixation as done during open surgery. Clips have the chance of slipping or abnormal migration later in life [2]. This is discussed more in detail in Chap. 12 (Video 6.2).

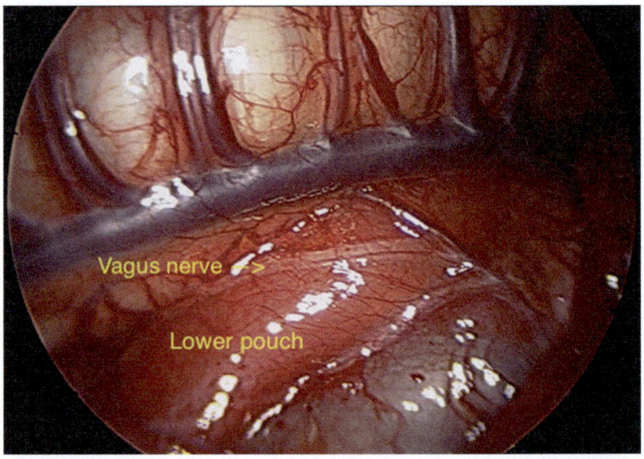

Fig. 6.3 Image showing identification of the lower pouch. Note the vagus nerve and the distended pouch insufflating with ventilation

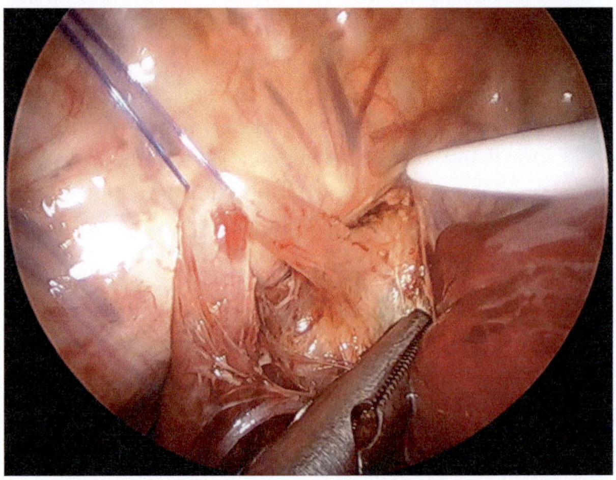

Fig. 6.4 Image showing the lower pouch looped by a prolene suture and lifted up with hitch to the chest wall

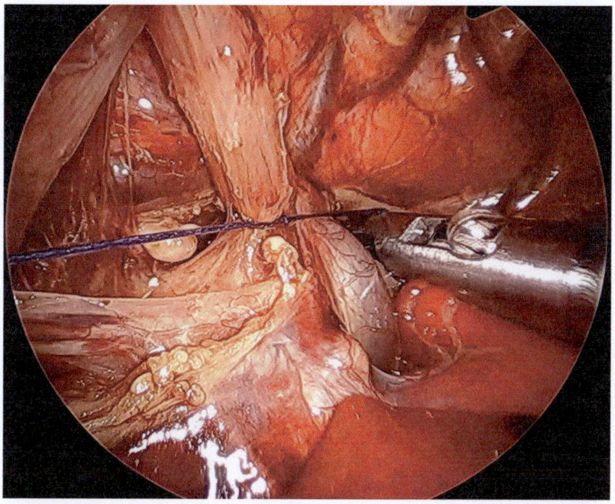

Fig. 6.5 Fistula being transfixed with suture at the level of tracheoesophageal junction

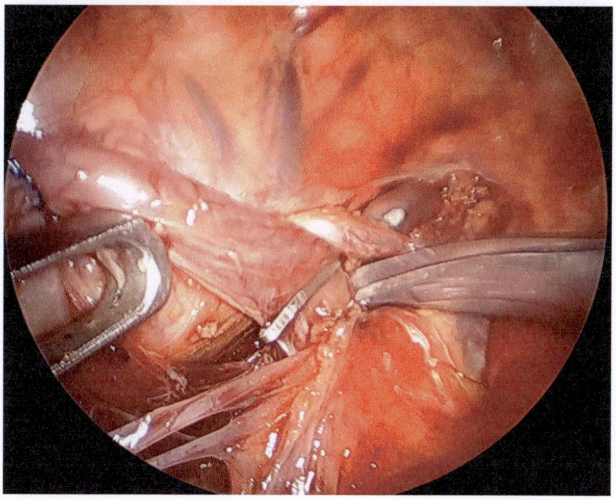

Fig. 6.6 Fistula with clip at the tracheoesophageal junction. Use of clip or suture to transfix is surgeon's preference

6.4 Upper Pouch Mobilization

Upper pouch mobilization is no different from what is done in open surgery. The endothoracic fascia is incised with hook cautery. A rigid tube is orally inserted in the upper pouch and is made to push forward by the anesthetist. This helps to identify the upper pouch by its movement. The upper pouch is grabbed with an atraumatic grasper and dissected circumferentially. It is of paramount importance to separate the upper pouch from trachea medially. This helps to gain length for a tension-free anastomosis along with exclusion of an upper pouch fistula. The dissection in the tracheoesophageal grove is a mix of sharp and blunt dissection (Fig. 6.7; Video 6.3).

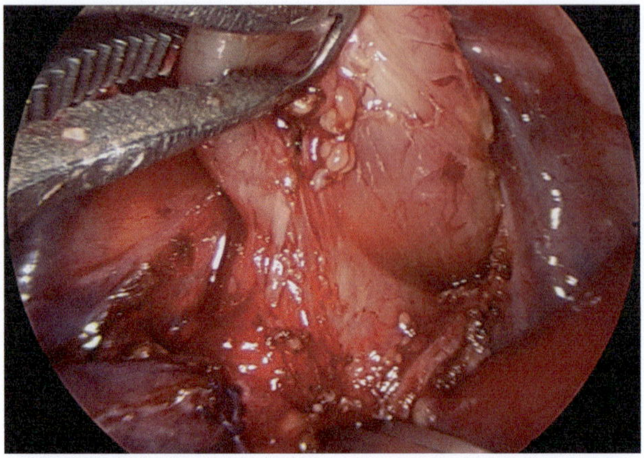

Fig. 6.7 The upper pouch is lifted with a grasper to show dissection plane between the esophagus and the trachea

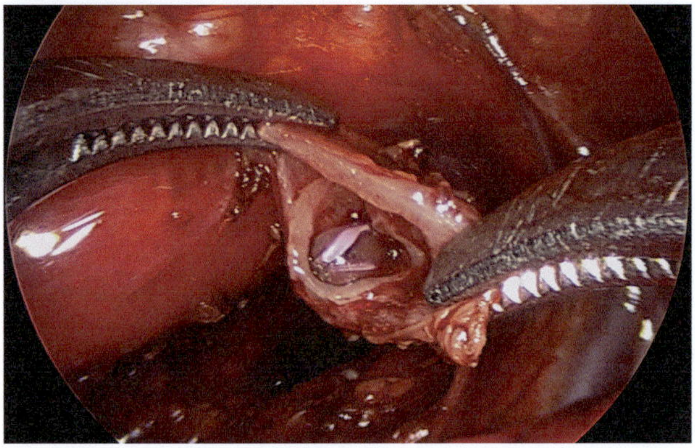

Fig. 6.8 Upper pouch completely mobilized with opened lumen. Note the retracted mucosal layer

A good pair of scissors is helpful, and it is advisable not to use sharp-tip scissors. Inadvertent tracheal injury is a possibility at this stage, and if this happens, it needs to be sutured with proline. Identification of correct plane between the trachea and esophagus is the key to avoid injury to either structure during dissection. It is worth mentioning that in authors' experience, the lower, the pouch is, the greater is the difficulty in separating it from the tracheal side as there is a longer common wall component. So, one should not underestimate the difficulty of dissection if the pouch is too low. In situations of difficult dissection, it is preferable to stay closer to esophagus than to the tracheal wall, as an inadvertent tracheal rent can have catastrophic consequences and at times very difficult to repair in a situation where the saturation may be falling due to ineffective ventilation.

Once the upper pouch is mobilized to satisfaction, an oblique cut is made in the dome of the pouch. This pouch is now ready for anastomosis. It may be noted that once the upper pouch is fully mobilized, the pouch becomes more and more retractile towards the thoracic inlet. The apparent gap may look higher at this stage, but a well-mobilized pouch will easily travel toward the anastomosis without much tension. Also, once the tip of upper pouch is opened, the mucosa retracts inward (Fig. 6.8). This is important while taking suture bites for anastomosis.

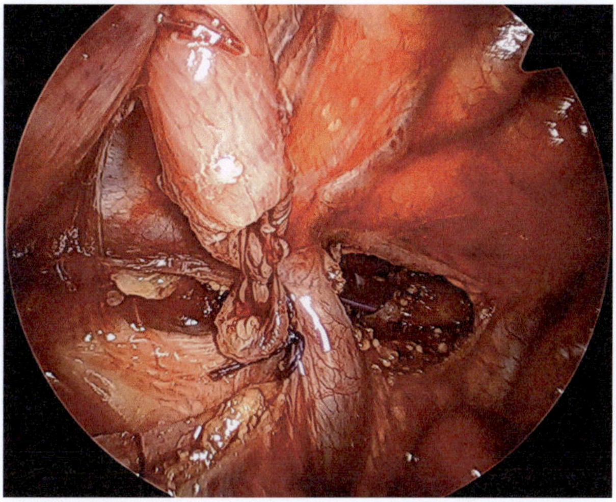

Fig. 6.9 Division of the ligated tracheoesophageal fistula. Note the partial division before the placement of first suture to avoid retraction

6.5 Preparing the Lower Pouch for Anastomosis

The lower pouch is now again lifted with the chest wall hitch and is divided in 2/3rd of the circumference leaving it still attached to the fistula (Fig. 6.9). Some surgeons will divide the ligated fistula completely. With complete division the lower pouch retracts toward the diaphragm and shrivels in size and length making the gap look more than it actually is. Partial division keeps the esophageal margins of lower end at the level of fistula and prevents any rotation during anastomosis. Once the first stitch is in place, the lower pouch can be completely disconnected and knot for first stitch is tied. This step may vary as per individual surgeon.

6.6 Handling Azygos Vein

Conventionally the azygos vein is ligated to facilitate the upper and lower pouch ligation. However, it has been shown that the azygos vein can be spared. This helps in better venous drainage of the lower pouch and lesser anastomotic edema [3]. The vein can be given gentle retraction with an additional suture hitch to move it out of the way of the pouches. The surgeon must plan how he intends to handle the azygos vein. This can be done by suture ligation (Fig. 6.10) or with the use of energy source. The anastomosis should be done medial and posterior to the azygos vein (Video 6.4).

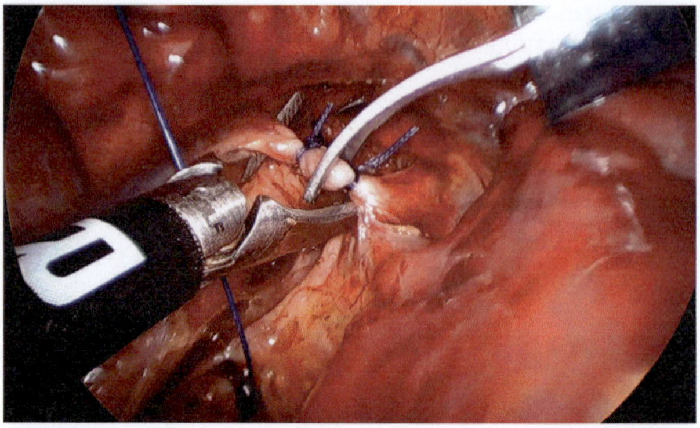

Fig. 6.10 Image showing division of azygos vein. The vein can be ligated and divided or can be handled with an energy source like harmonic scalpel

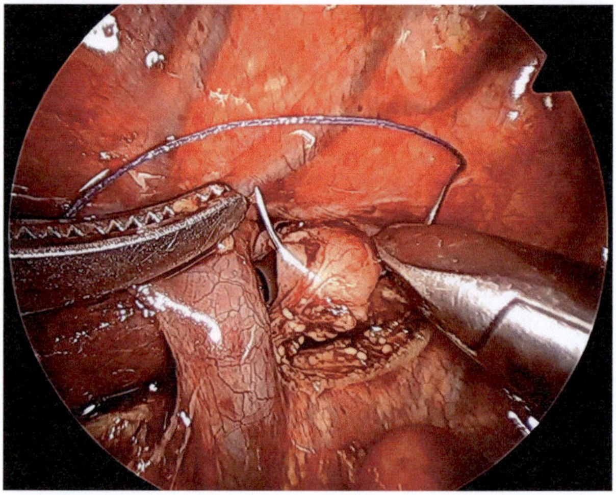

Fig. 6.11 Suture bite ensuring mucosa is taken in each anastomosis stitch

6.7 Anastomosis and the First Stitch

It is noteworthy that the placement of first stitch is important and difficult. The two esophageal ends tend to move away from each other, and the surgeon must ensure proper approximation and orientation. Bites are taken from the posterior wall segments of both the upper and lower pouches, and knot is preferably placed outside the lumen including the mucosa. It is mandatory to make sure that mucosa is taken in every bite (Fig. 6.11). The preferred suture is 5/0 vicryl with a half circle round body needle. The j-shaped needle which is hard to get can also be used if available. The first knot is done with a square triple throw to avoid loosening of knot. With a triple-throw knot, it is important to orient the free thread and the needle side thread in correct direction so that the knot is easily tightened. Pulling the threads in opposite orientation will do an improper tightening of the knot and will require greater

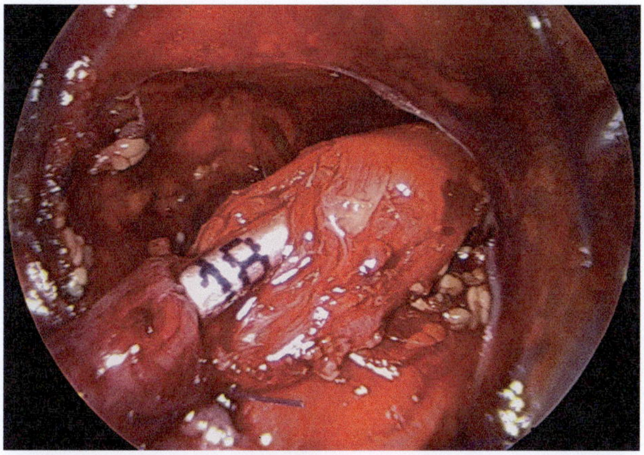

Fig. 6.12 Image showing the correct level of placement of trans-anastomotic tube with no. 18 visible in the field

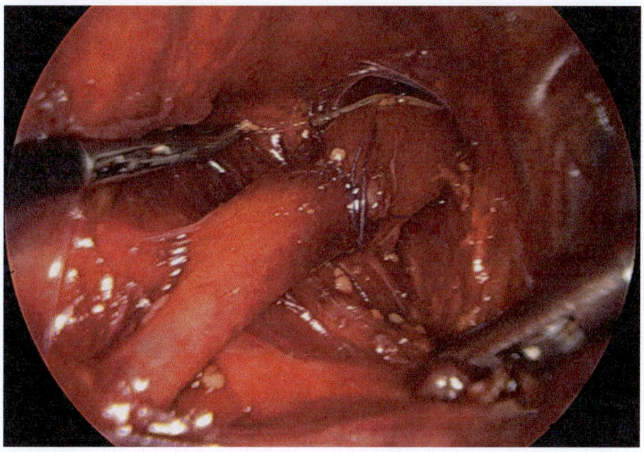

Fig. 6.13 Completed anastomosis with azygos division

force which can break the suture or cause bite through from the esophageal edges (Video 6.5).

Once the posterior layer is done, a size 6 Fr feeding tube is passed in the stomach as a trans-anastomotic tube and will be used as a feeding portal. It frequently happens that the tube passed from the nostril gets coiled in the oropharynx, and this is later realized at the end of the procedure. To avoid this the tube is held by the Maryland grasper, and the anesthetist is asked to give a tug to straighten the tube between the nostril and the anastomosis. This may be done more than once till one sees number 18 marking on the feeding tube (Fig. 6.12). This will be the final position of the tube with no coiling in oral cavity. The anastomosis is then completed, and at most five to six sutures are required in the entire anastomosis (Fig. 6.13 shows anastomosis with spared azygos, and Fig. 6.14 shows completed esophageal anastomosis with ligated azygos vein).

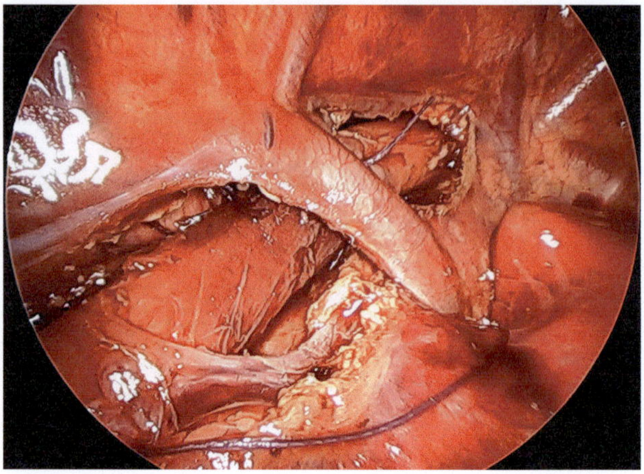

Fig. 6.14 Completed anastomosis with azygos sparing

6.8 Concluding the Operation

Once the anastomosis is done, the area is washed with saline. This also helps to check any air leaks and inadvertent tracheal injury. The anastomotic area is drained by a 12/14 Fr chest tube with underwater seal drain. The ports should be closed with rib approximation. The optical port is the best port to place the chest tube, but it is important to note that this port site is a straight punch hole in a thin chest wall. This does not provide a snug entry for the tube in the chest wall. This site will not collapse normally at the time of removal of the tube, and there is the possibility of pneumothorax if there is accidental dislodgement or removal of the chest tube. It is always better to take a closure stitch around the chest tube to make the entry snug and approximating. The incision sites are infiltrated with local anesthesia, and patient is handed over to the anesthesia team. The patient is then turned supine carefully being extremely cautious about the trans anastomotic and the chest tube.

6.9 Perioperative Care

The baby can be extubated if feasible and may or may not require ventilatory support. Feeding via trans-anastomotic tube can be started after 24 h in small volumes with gradual increments. Sequential chest X-rays are done as and when needed to monitor respiratory recovery, and the rest of the management is as per intensive care protocol. Most centers practice a contrast esophagogram after first week of surgery and will start on oral feeds if there is no leak. A follow-up esophagogram may be done at 3 months to look for stricture and need for dilatation.

6.10 Conclusion

To conclude thoracoscopic repair of esophageal atresia repair for classic type is a replica of the open procedure. The steps are the same except for thoracotomy. The avoidance of thoracotomy is a major benefit to the neonate and gives the benefit of faster recovery. The surgeon should be well versed with the open procedure to handle the steps and identify the anatomy.

References

1. McGowan NA, Grosel J. An overview of esophageal atresia and tracheoesophageal fistula. JAAPA. 2022;35(6):34–7. https://doi.org/10.1097/01.JAA.0000830180.79745.b9. PMID: 35617475.
2. Bindi E, Torino G, Noviello C, Simonini A, Torre M, D'Agostino R, Cobellis G. Recurrent tracheoesophageal fistula secondary to clips migration after thoracoscopic esophageal atresia repair. J Pediatr Surg Case Rep. 2020;62:101651.
3. Sharma S, Sinha SK, Rawat JD, Wakhlu A, Kureel SN, Tandon R. Azygos vein preservation in primary repair of esophageal atresia with tracheoesophageal fistula. Pediatr Surg Int. 2007;23(12):1215–8.

Suggested Reading

Kanojia R. Thoracoscopic repair of esophageal atresia. You Tube; 2017. https://youtu.be/AhVactADAgg?si=bsqrZiX-mbeGWmOw.

Kanojia R. Thoracoscopic repair of esophageal atresia (unedited video). You Tube; 2020. https://youtu.be/CpZrisvHKWc?si=7kkufVt0O6YEx_h7.

Kanojia R. Upper pouch dissection in TREAT. You Tube; 2021. https://youtu.be/4U25E-1xKyw?si=tc0p2rz5PgTGkwcY.

Thoracoscopic repair of esophageal atresia with tracheo-esophageal atresia. SpringerLink. n.d. https://link.springer.com/video/10.1007/978-981-99-3624-3.

Right Aortic Arch and Esophageal Atresia: Understanding the Anatomy and Approach

7

Contents

Learning Objectives

1. To understand the anatomy of right aortic arch in relation to esophageal atresia
2. Preoperative diagnosis
3. Approach right or left hemithorax
4. Thoracoscopic anatomy seen for right aortic arch during TREAT
5. Other vascular aberrations

Supplementary Information The online version contains supplementary material available at https://doi.org/10.1007/978-981-97-5695-7_7.

R. P. Kanojia, *Thoracoscopic Repair of Esophageal Atresia*,
https://doi.org/10.1007/978-981-97-5695-7_7

7.1 Introduction

Right aortic arch (RAA) and esophageal atresia is a rare combination of vascular and esophageal anomaly. The average incidence of esophageal atresia with RAA is roughly 5% of all esophageal atresia cases [1, 2]. The presence of abnormal arch on the right-side changes the anatomy even if the anatomy of esophageal atresia is of classic type. The surgical reconstruction becomes difficult, and the approach to the esophageal pouches varies with the presence of RAA. The right aortic arch has several variants, and other aberrations can be present along with RAA. With thoracoscopy the view is good enough to identify the anomaly intraoperatively. However, one must be aware of these anomalies to identify them correctly. This chapter deals with the basic anatomy of RAA in relation to esophageal atresia and answers some basic questions on the approach to such cases. Other common vascular aberrations are also discussed.

7.2 Embryology

The right aortic arch is a complex anomaly which is present in less than 1% of the population [3, 4]. The development of aortic arch is initiated as an aortic sac developing from truncus arteriosus. This arch then develops into the right and left horns. In normal development the right horn is absorbed as the brachiocephalic trunk, and the left horn becomes the part of arch giving rise to left subclavian and left common carotid. The two horns then continue into the right and left dorsal aorta (Fig. 7.1). In the abnormal development which ultimately develops into a right aortic arch, the left dorsal aorta is absorbed, and the right dorsal aorta persists resulting in a right aortic arch. Similarly, there can be a double aortic arch which is formed when both the dorsal aortas persist or have incomplete fusion.

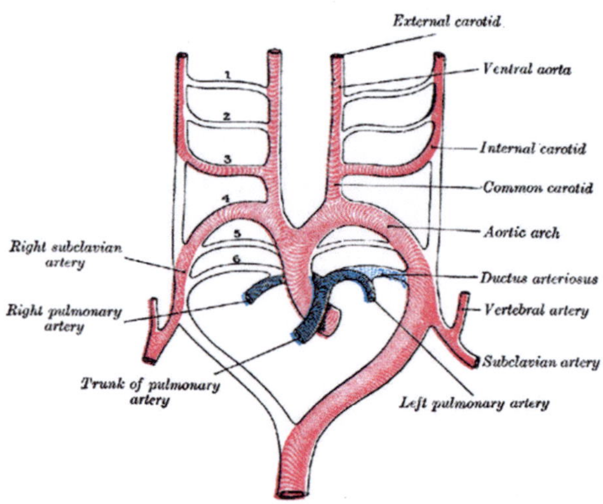

Fig. 7.1 Image showing the embryonic development of the aortic arches. The right horn is absorbed as the brachiocephalic trunk, and the left horn becomes the part of arch giving rise to left subclavian and left common carotid. (Image credit: Wikimedia commons)

7.3 Right Aortic Arch Anatomy

It is important to understand that the terminology of right and left in anatomical perspective is always in relation to a reference point. In the context of RAA, the reference point is the origin of the aorta from the left ventricle. In a normal instance, the arch arises from the left ventricle and loops to the left of its originating point and becomes the dorsal aorta. In RAA the arch loops to the right of the left ventricle and continues downward. In both instances the arch is to the left of midline and the vertebral column. Some literature will also mention that the normal arch goes behind the left bronchus and the RAA goes behind the right bronchus which is also true. There is a common misconception that the RAA or LAA is in reference to right or left of the vertebral column or the midline which is untrue.

The right aortic arch has three common types known as Types I, II, and III [5] (Fig. 7.2). The first variety is Type I, the mirror type (60% of all RAA). Here the vessels arising from the arch are mirror image of normal; i.e., the first branch is the left brachiocephalic trunk, and it is followed by the right common carotid and right subclavian.

The second variety (40%) is the variant where the first branch is left common carotid arising first, followed by the right common carotid, right subclavian, and then left subclavian arteries. Here the *left subclavian is the last branch* and is more on the right side must travel to the left side and usually loops around the esophagus resulting in an aberrant left subclavian artery vascular ring. This may produce esophageal compression symptoms. Type III is RAA with isolation of left subclavian artery. This is very rare and results from regression of segments of aortic arch proximal and distal to the origin of left subclavian vessel. Figure 7.3 shows the normal left aortic arch with its branches to compare the anatomy with the right arches.

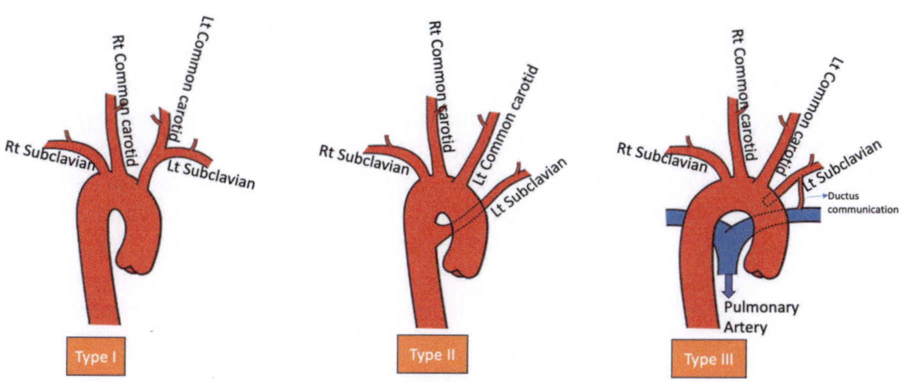

Fig. 7.2 Image showing three types of right aortic arches

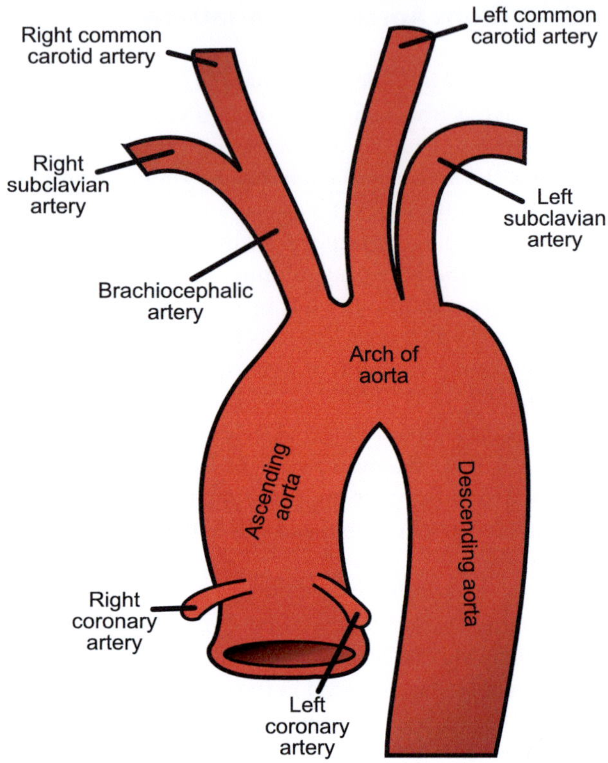

Fig. 7.3 Image showing the normal left aortic arch with its branches to compare the anatomy with the right arches

7.4 RAA and Esophageal Atresia

In the event of RAA coexisting with esophageal atresia and tracheoesophageal fistula, the anatomy becomes difficult for esophageal reconstruction as both the upper pouch and the fistula come to lie behind the arch and the descending aorta. This poses a dissection challenge during open and thoracoscopic surgery. The arch portion of the aorta overlies the upper esophageal pouch, and the descending part lies over the lower esophagus and fistula. The azygos vein arches over the descending part of the aorta. The preoperative diagnosis is difficult, and this is often seen as intraoperative surprise. Inexperienced surgeon can mistake the descending aorta as the lower esophagus. In the presence of the large pulsating aorta, the dissection of the upper and lower pouches is quite adventurous and can have serious vascular injuries. Of the two variants described, the mirror image variant is easier of the two

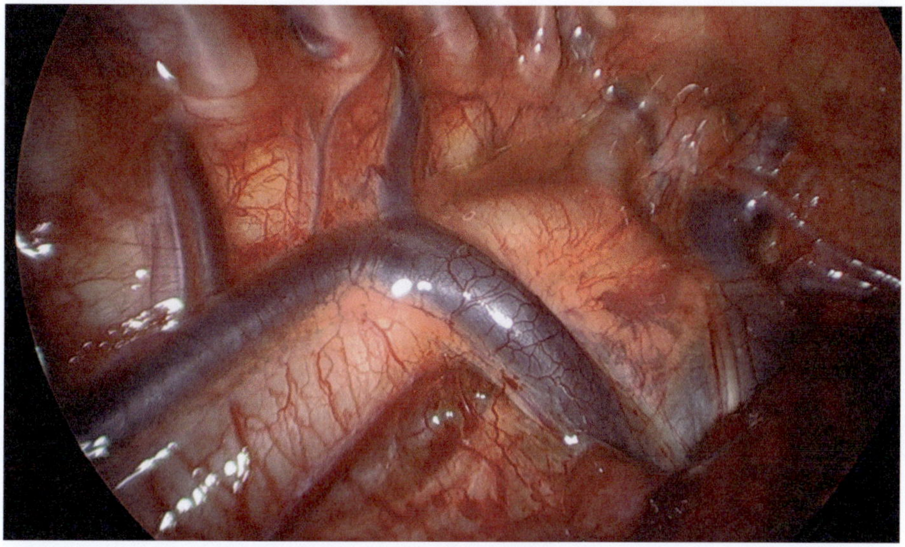

Fig. 7.4 Thoracoscopic view for EA-TEF and with RAA. Note how the aorta is prominently seen in the view

as there are no looping vessels over the upper pouch. Figure 7.4 shows the detailed thoracoscopic view for a normal esophageal atresia with tracheo-esophageal fistula (EA-TEF) and with RAA. Note how the aorta is prominently seen in the view (Video 7.1).

7.5 Preoperative Recognition

Echocardiographic evaluation is a part of all EA-TEF workup before surgery. Even with the best of efforts, the RAA and the vascular anomalies around the arch are difficult to identify. On preoperative chest X-ray, some patients may show an abnormal aortic knuckle on the right side (Fig. 7.5) raising a suspicion of an arch anomaly. This should further prompt for a detailed echocardiographic examination. In a series by Allan SR [6] of all patients with RAA, only 62.5% of RAA were diagnosed preoperatively by echocardiography, implying difficulty in characterizing the arch in a small neonate. Computed tomography (CT) angiogram is one of the best modalities to diagnose the vascular anomalies [7]. This can be safely done in newborn infants who are stable. MRI can provide similar imaging but requires

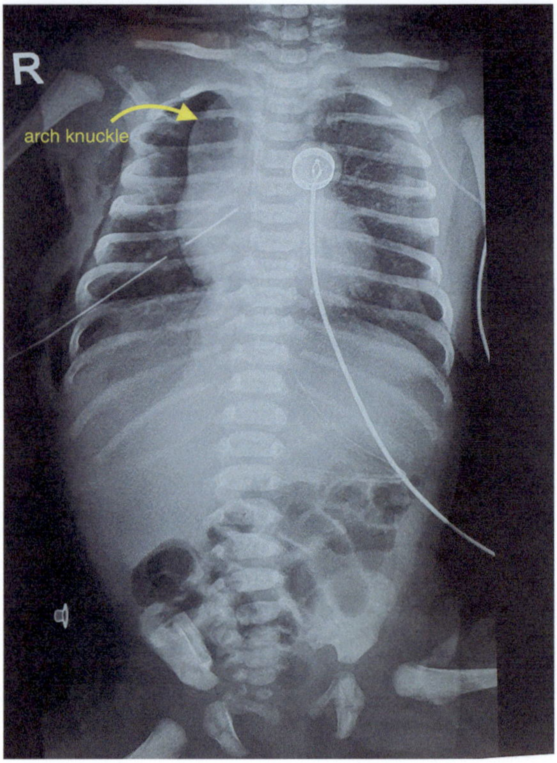

Fig. 7.5 Preoperative chest X-ray showing an abnormal aortic knuckle on the right side (arrow) raising a suspicion of an arch anomaly. This should further prompt for a detailed echocardiographic examination

anesthesia and long gantry time to complete the study making it less feasible in the preoperative period.

7.6 Right Versus Left Thoracotomy for EA-TEF with RAA

There is speculation in literature over the approach of conventional right versus left thoracic approach for the correction of EA-TEF. In order to have a satisfactory answer for this, it is first important to understand that majority of cases are undiagnosed preoperatively (only one in four is detected on a preoperative echocardiogram). For the small fraction of patients with confirmed diagnosis of RAA, a planned left thoracotomy is appropriate. The left thoracotomy provides easy exposure to the upper pouch and the fistula. It also prevents injury to the looping recurrent laryngeal nerve which will not be visible from the right approach.

For the cases when the preoperative information is not available and by default right approach is chosen, the decision to proceed intraoperatively depends on the ease of dissection, and surgeon must avoid any major mobilization of the aortic trunk or its branches. If the pouches are not found, the minimum target in such instance is to only ligate the fistula. A decision can be taken to do a left thoracotomy either in the same sitting or as a delayed procedure. A delayed procedure will provide an opportunity to evaluate the cardiac anomaly in detail, and a CT angiogram

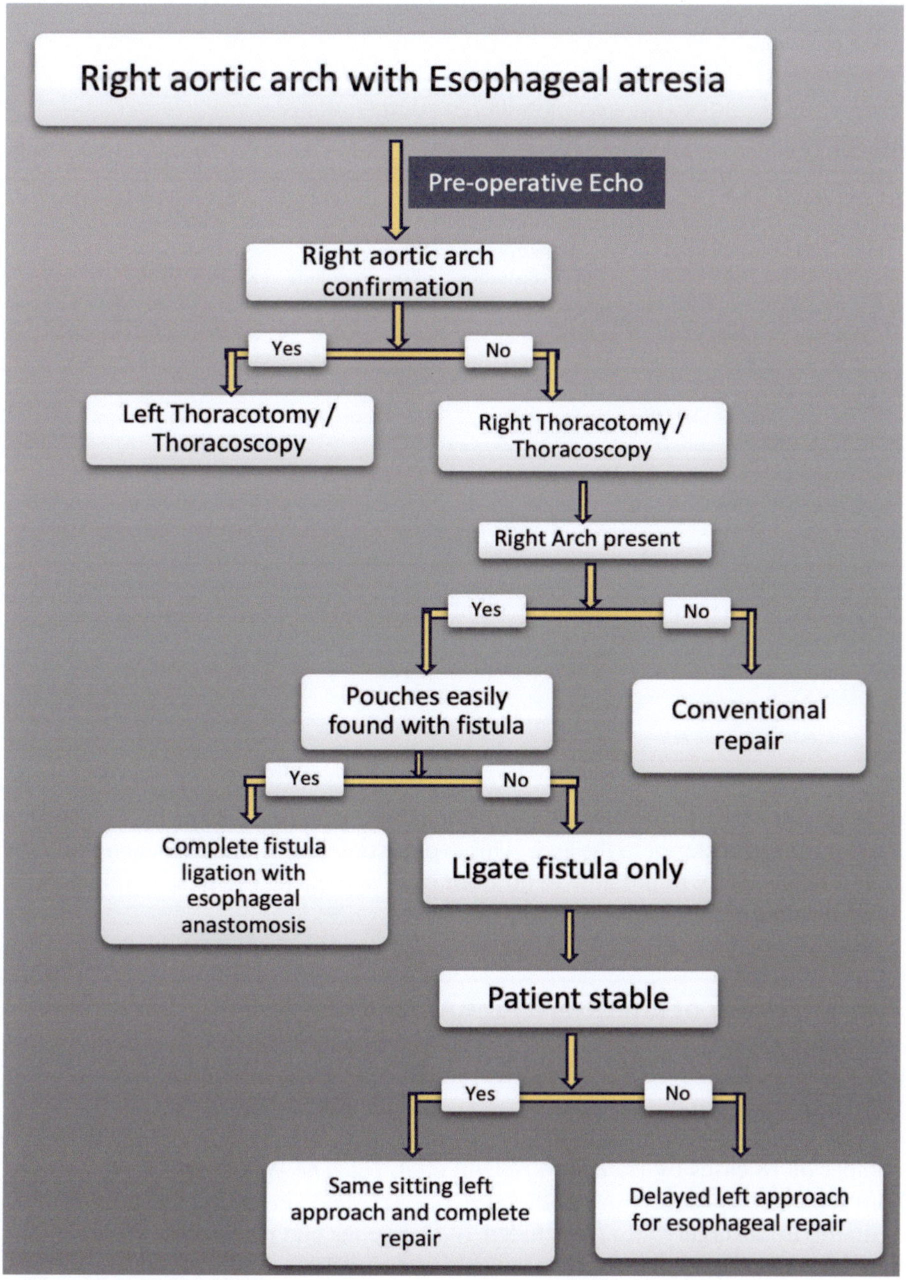

Fig. 7.6 Clinical decision-making algorithm for right aortic arch with esophageal atresia

Table 7.1 Summary of the major series of patients with esophageal atresia with RAA, reported in recent literature

S no	Author/year	Number of patients with RAA	Open/ thoracoscopic	Remarks
1.	Unal Bicakci et al. [8] (Turkey) 2009	11/79 (13%)	Open	Did right thoracotomy in all patients regardless of echo findings
2.	Filippo Parolini et al. [9] (Italy) 2015	Systematic review 8 studies with 54 patients	Open (3 thoracoscopic)	Pre-op detection in 7. Right 3. Left 4
3.	Steven R. Allen et al. (USA) 2006 [6]	8/61	Open	5/8 arch was correctly identified pre-op. 5 RT and 3 LT
4.	Rayuta Saka et al. [10] Japan 2020	One case	Thoracoscopic	Left thoracoscopy
5.	Kenneth K Y Wong [11] 2010 (Hong Kong)	2	Thoracoscopic	Pre-op information available about RAA still operated from right side
6.	Hamed M. Seleim et al. [1] (Egypt) 2022	18/121	Thoracoscopic	4/18 diagnosed pre-op. All right-side approach
7.	Babu R et al. [12] 1999 (London)	12/476	Open	11/12 right approach
8.	Dave R. Lal et al. 2018 (USA)	20/396	Open	12/20 right thoracotomy, 5 left side, 3 were long-gap atresia

or MRI can be done for further evaluation. The ideal location for the esophageal anastomosis is posterior to the arch. This avoids stretching of the esophagus over the arch. This is nearly impossible to do from right approach. The attached figure outlines the algorithm for the approach (Fig. 7.6).

7.7 Review of Literature for RAA with EA-TEF

Several series have been reported in literature about this combination Table 7.1 provides a summary of the major series reported in recent literature.

There are very few reports of thoracoscopic approach for RAA with the largest number of 18 cases by Hamed M Seleim et al. [1]. The side of approach is mixed with repair being done from both sides. A published survey by the International Pediatric Endosurgery Group included 144 surgeons and reported that over all left thoracoscopy should be the preferred approach for RAA with a clear diagnosis on pre-op echo. Thoracoscopy was found to be advantageous for these patients with a less aggressive approach.

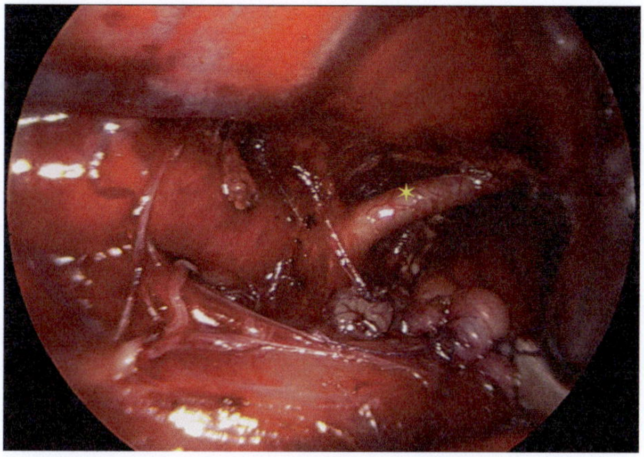

Fig. 7.7 Aberrant right subclavian artery (ARSA) seen next to the upper pouch

7.8 Thoracoscopic Anatomy for RAA with EA-TEF (Comparison with the Normal Thoracoscopic Anatomy)

Figure 7.4 shows the anatomical difference between normal arch and RAA in patients with EA-TEF. The upper pouch in the RAA is hidden behind the arch and is to be retrieved from the lower border of the arch. Similarly, the lower esophageal pouch and the fistula are also covered by the descending aorta. Video 7.2 demonstrates the thoracoscopic repair of EA-TEF with a RAA.

7.9 Other Vascular Aberrations

Apart from RAA there can be other vascular aberrations which can be seen as an intraoperative surprise. Aberrant right subclavian artery (ARSA) with a normal arch is another rare but more common among vascular anomalies seen with esophageal atresia. This has an incidence of approximately 12% among all the vascular aberrations [13]. Majority of these patients are diagnosed after the primary esophageal atresia surgery in the early neonatal period. The aberrant vessel causes compression over the esophagus and may result in dysphagia. Intraoperative recognition of this aberration is difficult but possible if the surgeon is aware of its existence. The vessel can be seen as a pulsating structure lateral to the upper pouch toward the vertebrae (Fig. 7.7). It is arising from the arch and going toward the left side. This vessel will cause an indentation on the upper esophagus and is seen in contrast esophagograms done in follow-up. Stephanie Berthet et al. [13] in a series of 254 upper Gastro-intestinal studies reported esophageal indentation in 7 which were confirmed to be ARSA. They concluded that the sensitivity and specificity of the upper GI contrast study are 66% and 98%, respectively. There is also a common association of long gap with esophageal atresia and the presence of other cardiac anomalies like tetralogy of Fallot.

7.10 Conclusions

The right aortic arch complicates the esophageal atresia repair. Surgical repair of esophageal atresia with RAA requires experience and knowledge of anatomy. With complete information available preoperatively, the left hemithorax is the preferred approach. In cases with the right approach, the intraoperative diagnosis the algorithm provided is to be followed. Surgeon should be familiar with the basics of the arch anomalies so that intraoperative findings can be properly recognized. Other common vascular aberrations like ARSA and ALSA should not be missed and should be looked for in case of abnormal anatomy. These can also be diagnosed after surgery in follow-up if the upper GI esophagogram is carefully evaluated and symptoms of dysphagia are followed up.

References

1. Seleim HM, Wishahy AMK, Magdy B, Elseoudi M, Zakaria RH, Kaddah SN, et al. The dilemma after an unforeseen aortic arch anomalies at thoracoscopic repair of esophageal atresia: is curtailing surgery still a necessity? Scand J Surg. 2022;111(2):14574969221090487.
2. Lal DR, Gadepalli SK, Downard CD, Minneci PC, Knezevich M, Chelius TH, et al. Infants with esophageal atresia and right aortic arch: characteristics and outcomes from the Midwest Pediatric Surgery Consortium. J Pediatr Surg. 2019;54(4):688–92.
3. Zidere V, Tsapakis EG, Huggon IC, Allan LD. Right aortic arch in the fetus. Ultrasound Obstet Gynecol. 2006;28(7):876–81.
4. Oztunc F, Ugan Atik S, Dedeoglu R, Yuksel MA, Madazli R. Aortic arch anomalies detected in foetal life by echocardiography. J Obstet Gynaecol. 2018;38(5):647–51.
5. Goel A, Viswamitra S. Congenital anomalies of aortic arch: a pictorial essay. Indian J Radiol Imaging. 2022;32(3):372–80.
6. Allen SR, Ignacio R, Falcone RA, Alonso MH, Brown RL, Garcia VF, et al. The effect of a right-sided aortic arch on outcome in children with esophageal atresia and tracheoesophageal fistula. J Pediatr Surg. 2006;41(3):479–83.
7. Katz M, Konen E, Rozenman J, Szeinberg A, Itzchak Y. Spiral CT and 3D image reconstruction of vascular rings and associated tracheobronchial anomalies. J Comput Assist Tomogr. 1995;19(4):564–8.
8. Bicakci U, Tander B, Ariturk E, Rizalar R, Ayyildiz SH, Bernay F. The right-sided aortic arch in children with esophageal atresia and tracheo-esophageal fistula: a repair through the right thoracotomy. Pediatr Surg Int. 2009;25(5):423–5.
9. Parolini F, Armellini A, Boroni G, Bagolan P, Alberti D. The management of newborns with esophageal atresia and right aortic arch: a systematic review or still unsolved problem. J Pediatr Surg. 2016;51(2):304–9.
10. Saka R, Tazuke Y, Ueno T, Nomura M, Deguchi K, Okuyama H. Esophageal atresia with right aortic arch: an experience of thoracoscopic repair through left thorax. Asian J Endosc Surg. 2021;14(2):301–4.
11. Wong KK, Tam PK. Thoracoscopic repair of esophageal atresia through the right chest in neonates with right-sided aortic arch. J Laparoendosc Adv Surg Tech A. 2010;20(4):403–4.
12. Babu R, Pierro A, Spitz L, Drake DP, Kiely EM. The management of oesophageal atresia in neonates with right-sided aortic arch. J Pediatr Surg. 2000;35(1):56–8.
13. Berthet S, Tenisch E, Miron MC, Alami N, Timmons J, Aspirot A, et al. Vascular anomalies associated with esophageal atresia and tracheoesophageal fistula. J Pediatr. 2015;166(5):1140–4.e2.

Conversion to Open, Intraoperative Complications and Management During TREAT (Vascular Injury/Tracheal Injury)

8

Contents

Learning Objectives

1. Reasons for converting to open procedure
2. Injury to trachea and its management
3. Vascular injury during TREAT

Supplementary Information The online version contains supplementary material available at https://doi.org/10.1007/978-981-97-5695-7_8.

R. P. Kanojia, *Thoracoscopic Repair of Esophageal Atresia*, https://doi.org/10.1007/978-981-97-5695-7_8

8.1 Introduction

Conversion to open (CTO) is a part of any minimal access procedure. It should not be considered a complication if the primary objective is achieved. In the initial part of a learning curve, the need for conversion can be multifactorial, and the surgeon alone is not the only variable. There is a complex interplay between the surgeon, the camera assistant, and the anesthetist. The camera assistant and the anesthetist play a crucial role in the procedure's success. The camera person should be well versed in small space optics and ergonomics to give the surgeon the best possible view. Ventilating the lung is the biggest hurdle for the camera person to provide target area visibility to the surgeon. Similarly, an anesthetist must synchronize with the operative steps, allowing room for the surgeon. Lack of harmony between the three can cause difficulties and patient instability, leading to conversion. This chapter describes various team and patient-related factors responsible for conversion to open and possible ways to circumvent the problems.

8.2 Intraoperative Causes for Conversion

8.2.1 Loss of Working Space Due to Ventilating Lung

At the beginning of the procedure, the anesthetist is ventilating the baby who has just been turned to a right lateral/semi-prone position. The anesthetist will use higher end expiratory pressures to maintain neonatal saturation. This will result in persistent hyperinflation of the right lung and loss of working space for the surgeon. The surgeon initially tackles the situation by establishing a positive CO_2 pressure of 4–5 mmHg. This will result in desaturation. In unfavorable situations there will be multiple episodes of desaturation forcing the surgeon to deflate the chest and wait till the saturation picks up. Even when the saturation picks up and surgeon is back in the chest, he is unable to get a working space due to an inflating lung. If this continues for long, there will be poor vision, repeated fogging, and no progress in the steps of surgery. In such situation a collective decision is needed between the anesthetist and the surgeon on whether to proceed with thoracoscopy or convert to open (Video 8.1).

There are several possible reasons for given situation. Most important is a poorly optimized patient. Any neonate with bad lungs especially evidence of pneumonia on the left side will maintain poorly in the right lateral position where the good left lung is dependent and is poorly perfused and ventilated.

8.2.2 Use of High Pressure

Undue use of high thoracic CO_2 pressure will result in compression of the superior vena cava and reduction of preload in the heart which will set a cycle of poor ventilation perfusion of both lungs. This will be evident with the immediate pickup of

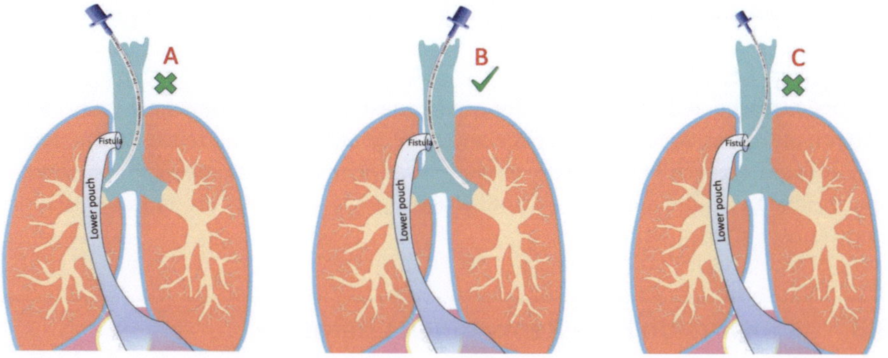

Fig. 8.1 Image showing the three different positions of endotracheal tube that can occur after intubation. (**b**) is the correct desired position. (**a**) and (**c**) will lead to difficult patient ventilation and higher chance of conversion

saturation after deflation. The surgeon can try to establish his working space with pressures as low as 3 mmHg to avoid desaturation.

8.2.3 Improper Intubation

The ideal intubation in a patient requiring TREAT is an endotracheal tube tip placed beyond the fistula with the bevel toward the left side so that full ventilation is achieved for the left lung with limited ventilation of the right lung and no air gets pushed toward the fistula. Neonatal intubation is difficult achieving this ideal state of the endotracheal tube is difficult. There are situations where the reverse happens when the tip of the endotracheal tube is close to the right bronchus and fistula. This will result in all pressures being delivered to the right lung, and there will be loss of working space for the surgeon, and it will be difficult for him to proceed with the steps of the surgery. Anesthesia and ventilation are discussed in detail in the relevant sections of this book. Figure 8.1 shows the three different positions of the endotracheal tube as described above.

8.2.4 Difficult Anatomy

Individual cases may have anatomical variations which are difficult to tackle thoracoscopically. The presence of vascular anomaly is the most common cause which can force for conversion. The right aortic arch aberrant looping subclavian artery are a common example of the vascular anomaly which makes the dissection of the upper pouch and the fistula difficult. More details about the right aortic arch are discussed in Chapter 7.

8.2.5 Long Gap and Inability to Anastomose

A long gap between the atretic ends is also a frequent reason to convert. In the authors experience thoracoscopic long-gap anastomosis of esophageal ends can be difficult at times due to limited space and limited suturing experience. In this condition, it is quite possible to achieve a hand-sewn primary anastomosis if converted to open. Hence it is the surgeon's discretion if he wants to convert and complete the anastomosis after opening.

8.3 Conversion Rate Reported in Literature

In a systematic review, Roberta V et al. [1] reported that the conversion rate was 9.6% (37/382) of the patients in the 14 series included in the meta-analysis. Of these 37 patients, 10 patients required conversion because of ventilation-related issues. Six patients had conversion because of knotting difficulties. Insufficient surgical exposure was the cause in four patients.

8.4 Intraoperative Complications

8.4.1 Tracheal Injury

Mobilization of the upper pouch is a crucial step to achieve tension-free anastomosis. In this step the more crucial part is the medial separation of the upper pouch from the tracheal wall. There is a common wall component between the lateral tracheal wall and the medial wall of the esophagus. The separation is to be done by a mix of sharp and blunt dissection, and once a proper plane is reached, the blunt dissection can separate the two walls and complete mobilization can be achieved. It has been commonly observed that, the lower the upper pouch is, the more difficult it is to separate it from the trachea. During separation if there is an accidental rent in the tracheal wall, then it must be dealt with immediately to prevent air leak. The best course of action in such situation is to know the site of the rent in relation to the tip of the endotracheal tube. If the endotracheal tube is proximal to the rent, then there will be more air leak and the patient can desaturate fast. In such situation the anesthetist can gently slide the endotracheal tube past the tracheal rent and keep ventilating. The rent can then be repaired using 5/0 prolene. Usually with small pinpoint rent, a simple figure of eight stitches will close the rent. For bigger longitudinal rent, a proper continuous suture line is needed.

An easy injury to the tracheal while mobilizing the upper pouch can be a sign of membranous tracheal wall and a possibility of tracheomalacia. This should prompt the surgeon to look for the visibility of tracheal rings and collapse of the trachea with the ventilation. This may require further intervention in the postoperative period ranging from tracheostomy to posterior tracheopexy as an additional procedure.

The reported incidence of tracheal injury is not known due to its infrequent occurrence. Patkowski et al. [2] reported two cases of tracheal injury out of 23 patients. Similarly, Paweł Nachulewicz et al. [3] reported 1 tracheal injury in his 10-patient series.

8.4.2 Vascular Injuries

The posterior mediastinum and thoracic inlet, where the upper pouch is located, are very busy areas. There are several large vessels which if injured can lead to exsanguinating bleeding. The problem with an ongoing bleeding and the use of suction to clear the area is that when a suction is used to aspirate blood, there is loss of pneumothorax and lungs immediately expand resulting in loss of working space and vision, making it difficult to control, and this can be one of the reasons for conversion to open.

The azygos vein is the first vascular structure and is usually divided either by suture ligation or using a vessel sealer. The azygos vein medially unites with the main trunk of the superior vena cava. Any slippage of ligature or bleeding due to improper sealing of the superior vena cava side of the vein can be catastrophic as there is short stump. The flow of bleeding will be high due to the proximity to the right atrium. Pressure application and precise gripping of the stump are important to control the bleeding. The ligation of the azygos vein is a simple step and should be done with due diligence.

Arterial injuries can happen to the subclavian vessels at the time of the upper pouch mobilization specially when there are arch anomalies present. Aberrant right subclavian vessel can be present in rare cases which arises from the arch and courses toward the left side. This vessel is present close to the lateral part of the upper pouch and can be injured while mobilizing it. Similarly, while mobilizing the lower pouch, the aorta itself or the small vertebral branches can be injured resulting in bleeding and be a cause of CTO. The threshold for conversion for such injuries should be low as the volume reserve in neonates is low and they will exsanguinate fast. The presence of aberrant right subclavian artery arising from the arch and running to the left side if not recognized during upper pouch mobilization will cause torrential bleeding. This is a rare anomaly seen in 9% of all vascular aberrations [4] seen in association with esophageal atresia.

Figure 8.2 represents the summation of all the possible causes for conversion to open described in the preceding text.

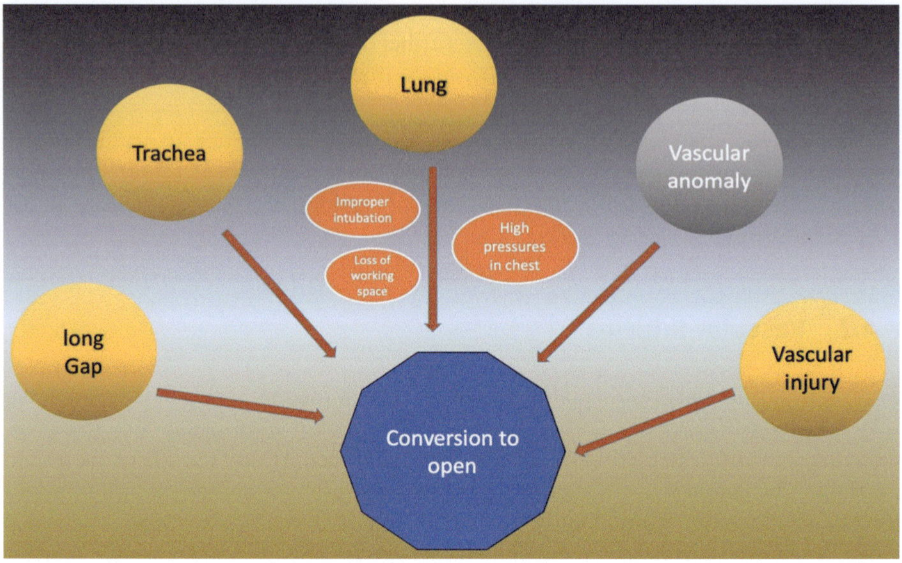

Fig. 8.2 Summation infographic of possible reasons for conversion to open during TREAT

8.5 Conclusions

Intraoperative complications and conversion to open in early and complex cases are part of the learning process. Conversion to open is higher in the earlier set of cases, and as the team's experience gets better, the surgeon's resilience to challenging scenarios increases, and he can handle complicated anatomy. The threshold for conversion to open should be low in an unstable patient. Preoperative patient stabilization and optimization are essential, and a fit neonate will tolerate the procedure easily, and outcomes will be better.

References

1. Iacona RV, Saxena AK. Thoracoscopic repair of esophageal atresia with distal tracheoesophageal fistula (type C): systematic review. Surg Laparosc Endosc Percutan Tech. 2020;30(4):388–93.
2. Patkowsk D, Rysiakiewicz K, Jaworski W, Zielinska M, Siejka G, Konsur K, et al. Thoracoscopic repair of tracheoesophageal fistula and esophageal atresia. J Laparoendosc Adv Surg Tech A. 2009;19(Suppl 1):S19–22.
3. Nachulewicz P, Zaborowska K, Rogowski B, Kalinska A, Nosek M, Golonka A, et al. Thoracoscopic repair of esophageal atresia with a distal fistula—lessons from the first 10 operations. Wideochir Inne Tech Maloinwazyjne. 2015;10(1):57–61.
4. Berthet S, Tenisch E, Miron MC, Alami N, Timmons J, Aspirot A, et al. Vascular anomalies associated with esophageal atresia and tracheoesophageal fistula. J Pediatr. 2015;166(5):1140–4.e2.

9 Short-Term Complications and Management After TREAT

Contents

Learning Objectives

1. Perioperative complications and their management
2. Management of intraoperative leak
3. Indications for diversion

9.1 Introduction

Thoracoscopic repair of esophageal atresia is a complex and technically demanding procedure. There may be complications due to the technicalities of the procedure or due to the native anatomy. The previous chapter had discussed the possible intraoperative complications that can happen and how to manage them. Once the procedure is completed uneventfully, there is still a battle to be won in the early postoperative

---

Supplementary Information The online version contains supplementary material available at https://doi.org/10.1007/978-981-97-5695-7_9.

R. P. Kanojia, *Thoracoscopic Repair of Esophageal Atresia*,
https://doi.org/10.1007/978-981-97-5695-7_9

period, and success cannot yet be declared. There can be several complications that can happen in the early postoperative period. For the sake of convenience, the time of early complications is defined as any complication happening within 3 months of surgery and requiring intervention or which prolongs the hospital stay beyond the expected duration. This chapter aims to describe the complications occurring in the said period and their management with the evidence available from the literature. We will describe complications specific to thoracoscopy. Some part of the discussion will delve into the evidence in literature if these complication rates are different in open and thoracoscopic approach.

9.2 Complications

The entire spectrum of early complications can be divided into early complications immediately after surgery and early complications within 14 days to 3 months after surgery. These are described below.

9.2.1 Early Complications Immediately After Surgery (0–14 Postoperative Period)

1. Postoperative anastomotic leak
2. Air leak
3. Chylothorax

9.2.1.1 Postoperative Anastomotic Leak

Anastomotic leak is the most common complication which can occur immediately after surgery. The incidence of leak in general is reported as 10–20% [1, 2]. The appearance of leak can happen ranging from day 2 to day 6. Early leaks have a more chance of being a major leak. Generally, these patients are managed by observation, antibiotics, and parenteral nutrition, except in circumstances where leak is major and requires surgical intervention. The causes for leak are multifactorial. Anastomotic gap and resultant anastomotic tension are the most important factor which can predict leak and chances of resolution. The common causes of anastomotic leak are listed and described below.

Long Gap with Tension in Anastomosis

Long-gap atresia is the most common and accurate factor which can predict the occurrence of leak. In a study by Jin Xi Huang et al. [3], the chances of leak in long-gap atresia were 4.9 times higher than the non-long-gap atresia, and patients with >3 cm atresia were more prone to leak. The presence of long gap can be anticipated on the preoperative X-rays, and if there are other comorbidities like cardiovascular anomalies, preterm, low birth weight, etc., then the chances of having a leak will be higher. Surgical anastomosis in long gap warrants mobilization of esophageal pouches. As a priority the upper pouch is mobilized to the maximum extent. After

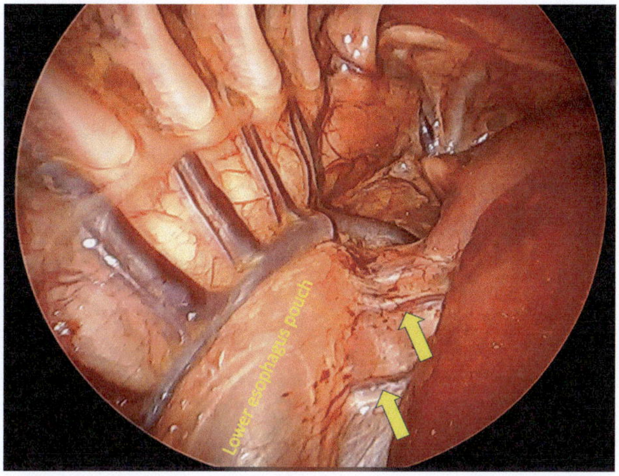

Fig. 9.1 Intraoperative image of undissected lower esophageal pouch showing the blood supply coming in perpendicular axis to the length of esophagus (arrows). These branches will be disrupted if the lower pouch is mobilized extensively

complete mobilization of the upper pouch, if anastomosis cannot be done, then the lower pouch is mobilized to bridge the gap. The blood supply to the lower pouch is tenuous and receives blood supply in the lateral perpendicular axis with branches from the bronchial side and branches from the aortic side. These branches are very small tenuous and are easily disrupted due to mobilization (Fig. 9.1). Once mobilized the vascularity of the end of the lower esophageal stump will depend on a submucosal supply via the lower part of the esophagus supplied by the inferior phrenic artery and the ascending branch of the left gastric artery. This is the reason; the lower esophagus stump will always look discolored after the completion of the anastomosis. Poor venous drainage with ischemia results in local site edema, dehiscence in the suture line, and leak. This phenomenon of leak due to vascular insult can happen independent of long gap. Patients with kissing pouch or short gap if subjected to extensive mobilization of upper and lower esophageal pouches can have leak even if there is no anastomotic tension. This explains the importance of preserving vascularity while handling the esophageal tissue. In classic esophageal atresia with tracheoesophageal fistula and long gap, every attempt should be made to achieve primary anastomosis. Taking a chance with extensive mobilization of esophageal pouches may sometimes be worthwhile if primary anastomosis is achieved. The issue of long gap and management in such cases is discussed in Chap. 11.

Technical Faults: Failure to Include Mucosa in All the Sutures

Esophageal anastomosis in thoracoscopy is challenging due to small working space and constant interruption by the moving lung. Once the upper pouch is mobilized, the pouch is opened over the tip of the feeding tube being pushed by the anesthetist. Once this is done and the upper pouch is open, the mucosa of the upper pouch somewhat recedes up in the opened lumen. The edge of the outer wall and the edge of mucosa are at different level (Fig. 9.2). This happens with all thick wall luminal structures with muscular coat and mucosa. Another example of a similar thing happening is with thick-walled urinary bladder. These bladders when opened for

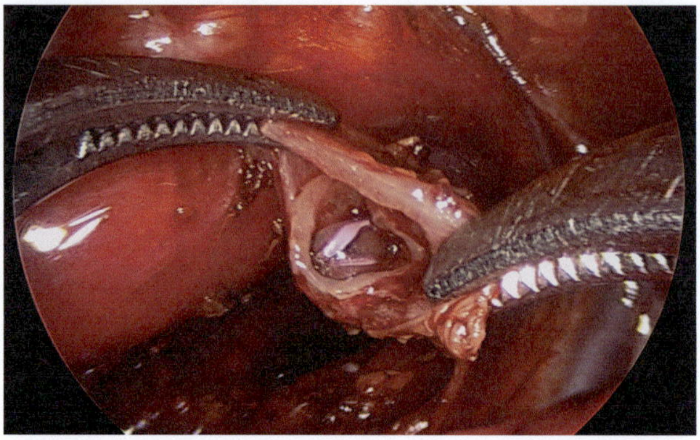

Fig. 9.2 Opened upper pouch with mucosa seen retracted into the lumen

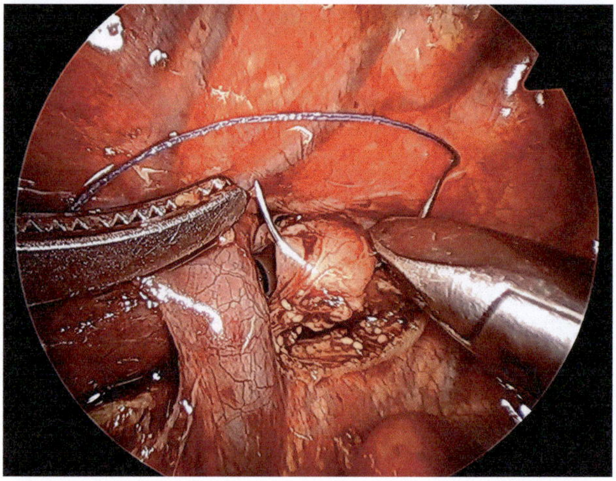

Fig. 9.3 Image showing anastomosis in progress with suture needle passing deep enough to take a bite of mucosa

vesicostomy the mucosa recedes and must be dragged out with every bite during vesicostomy. This does not happen with the lower pouch of the esophagus as it is thin walled. Surgeon must ensure that while doing the anastomosis mucosa is included in every bite of the upper pouch (Fig. 9.3), if not included the mucosal gap will lead to an anastomotic leak irrespective of gap or other factors listed above.

Anastomosis Around Vascular Anomalies Like RAA and Anomalous Vessels Leading to Stretching of Anastomosis

This is a relatively rare situation, and less than 10% of esophageal atresia undergoing primary anastomosis will have vascular anomalies like the right aortic arch and anomalous vessels around the upper pouch [4, 5]. The presence of anomalous arch seen as an intraoperative surprise will make anastomosis difficulty, and if the surgeon is able to do the anastomosis over the arch, there will be some tension as the esophagus is stretched over the arch which is constantly pulsating. This will lead to higher chance of anastomotic leak. This factor can be taken care of by having a good mobilization and tension-free anastomosis as far as possible. The right aortic arch is discussed in detail in Chap. 7.

Poor Patient Optimization Before and After Surgery with Sepsis, Low Albumin, and Poor Perfusion

Patient selection is crucial for thoracoscopic repair. The case selection criteria are discussed in Chap. 3. Even after selecting the best-case scenarios, it is important that the patient is optimized for surgery. A septic patient will have multi-organ dysfunction and poor central and peripheral perfusion. This becomes crucial in healing of an already precarious anastomosis due to other anatomical factors. A patient who is septic requiring inotropes will always have higher chances of anastomosis leak. Similarly, albumin levels are indicator of nutritional status of the neonate and have a direct impact on anastomotic side edema and healing. In a study by Jin Xi Huang et al. [3], low serum albumin levels were associated with higher leak rate in univariate analysis. This is conversely proven by the fact that most of the minor leaks are managed by nutritional support and majority resolve after parenteral nutrition and supportive management.

Indications of Diversion

Esophageal diversion after unresolving leak is done as a last resort for an unresolving major leak. Continued leak of saliva in the mediastinum will lead to mediastinitis, collapse of the right lung, and sepsis. The management of anastomotic leak after a thoracoscopic repair can be slightly different from a leak happening after a thoracotomy repair. With thoracoscopy the tolerance to the consequences of leak is better as the morbidity of thoracotomy is avoided. Moreover, if one has to re-open the chest, it will be the first thoracotomy for the newborn as opposed to the second for open cases. Two back-to-back thoracotomies in a short span of time for a newborn can be catastrophic. The indications of diversion after a thoracoscopic repair are no different from what is followed with open repairs. The first step in the management is the quantification of leak as major or minor. The algorithm for the management, approach, and indications for diversion if there is anastomotic leak is presented in Fig. 9.4. There have been some recent reports [1] of approaching leak repairs as redo thoracoscopy rather than opening chest with success. This is included in this algorithm.

9.2.1.2 Air Leak and Pneumothorax After Thoracoscopic Repair

After completion of thoracoscopic repair, a small percentage of patients may show air leak from the chest tube with pneumothorax. The possible causes of air leak can be the following:

1. *Air Leak from Minor Lung Injury*: The leak may be a result of minor lung injury occurring from handling of the right lung with laparoscopic instruments and causing parenchymal injuries. This if happens is usually minor and is self-limiting with no intervention required.
2. *Improper Ligation of Fistula* is rare and avoidable complication. This leads to air leak coming from improperly ligated fistula. When this happens, the leak is usu-

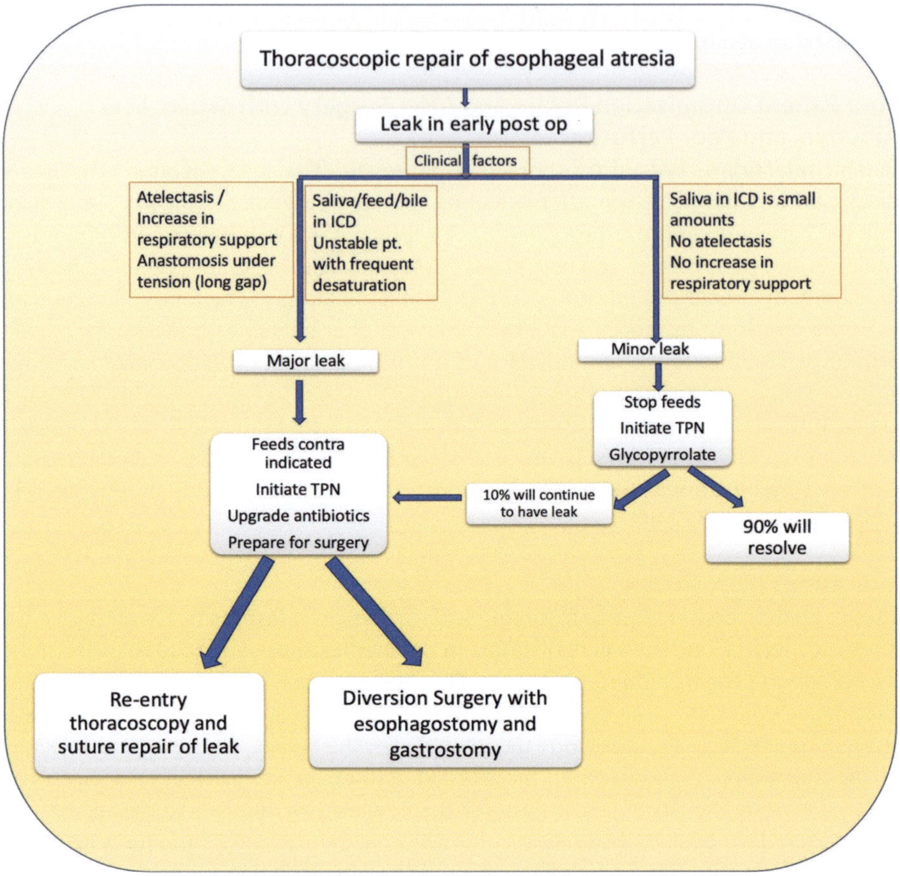

Fig. 9.4 Algorithm for management of leak in postoperative period. Note the option of reentry thoracoscopy and suture repair of leak

ally large and is synchronized with ventilation. The patient in this situation will be very unstable and will require re-exploration to deal with the fistula site. The chance of spontaneous resolution in such situations is very low.

3. *Pneumothorax with Anastomotic Leak and Mechanical Ventilation*: having an anastomotic leak in the early postoperative period when the neonate is still being ventilated will have a higher chance of developing pneumothorax. This happens because of air tracking down from the glottis to the esophagus and escaping into the mediastinum. In a study by Jiawei Zhao et al. [6] showed via a multivariate logistic regression analysis that postoperative anastomotic leakage and mechanical ventilation are independent risk factors for pneumothorax after esophageal atresia repair. This study included both open and thoracoscopic repair in equal proportions. His major part of the treatment involved pleural drainage and conservative management. In another study by M. Besendorfer et al. [7], a clear relation with anastomotic failure was established and concluded that that this may be the first sign of an anastomotic leak. Interestingly there are reports [8] that postopera-

tive patients who were extubated within few days of surgery had pneumothorax on the day of extubation, and this was realized soon that these patients after extubation were kept on high-flow nasal continuous positive airway pressure mode and this caused esophageal insufflation and air leak through the anastomotic area and resultant pneumothorax. The pneumothorax immediately resolved once the neonate was kept on hood oxygen and recovered completely.

9.2.1.3 Chylothorax

Chylothorax is a rare but known complication of mediastinal surgeries. Procedures involving mediastinal dissection will have a high chance of injuring the thoracic duct owing to the anatomy of the duct. Anatomically the duct begins as cisterna chyli at the level of T-12 vertebrae and courses parallel to the right side of the vertebral column. The duct enters the thorax through the aortic hiatus into the posterior mediastinum. The duct travels more to the right of the vertebrae behind the esophagus in the lower part of the posterior mediastinum and courses itself to the left side of the vertebral column before ending into the left subclavian adjacent to the left internal jugular confluence (Fig. 9.5). There is an additional right lymphatic duct which drains the right arm and upper chest regions and drains in to the right subclavian. Injury to these ducts can happen with extensive dissection to the posterior mediastinum and can result in chylothorax. During esophageal atresia surgery, the duct is more likely to be injured if there is extensive mobilization of the upper pouch

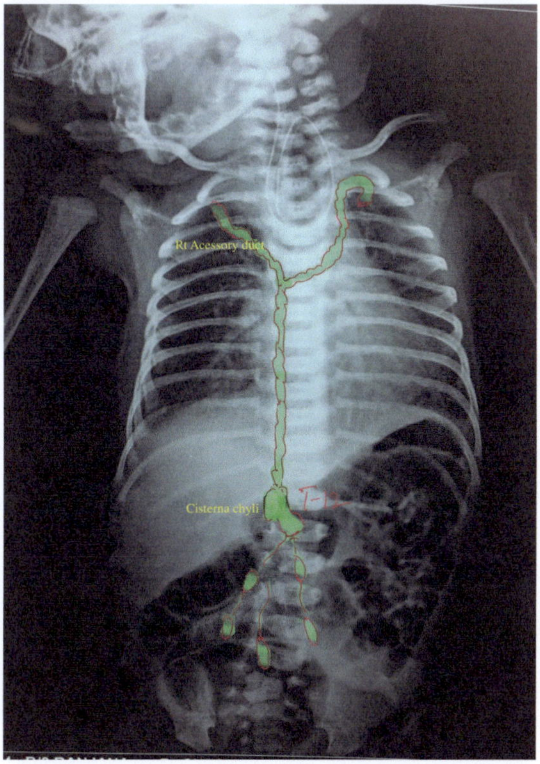

Fig. 9.5 Anatomy of thoracic duct projected over X-ray of EA-TEF patient. Note how the duct travels to the right of vertebral column and crosses to left side at the carina. The right accessory duct lies in close proximity to the upper pouch

or lower pouch. The upper pouch can injure the right accessory duct, and the lower pouch mobilization can injure the main thoracic duct. The tributaries of the duct also drain into the azygos vein, and improper division of the azygos vein can lead to leak from these tributaries.

To avoid injury to the lymphatic duct structures, it is advisable to have a clean ligation of the azygos vein. The dissection of the upper and lower pouch should be precise without any blunt dissection and traction on surrounding structures. Roy S et al. [9] suggested that majority of chylothorax leakage sites are near the azygos vein, and they suggested it to do a clean ligation rather than by vessel sealing or diathermy. He also reported the use of Indocyanine Green (ICG) imaging to visualize the thoracic duct to prevent the injury while doing esophageal dissection. He used ICG imaging in three cases of EA-TEF patients who had chylothorax after TREAT and detected the site of leakage by ICG imaging.

In general, the management of chylothorax is conservative with supportive treatment. Enteral feeding is stopped, and total parenteral nutrition is started with medium chain triglycerides. If this fails to resolve and output is high >100 ml/kg/day, then a second-line treatment somatostatin or octreotide is started with factor VIII infusion. Surgical intervention is the last line of management when there is no resolution. The surgical options include advanced options like ICG imaging and locating the site of leak. The other options are ligation of the duct if leak site is visible, pleurodesis with fibrin glue or pleuroperitoneal shunt.

9.2.2 Early Complications (14 Days to 3 Months After Surgery)

9.2.2.1 Re-fistulation or Recurrence of TEF

Recurrent TEF (rTEF) is a common complication after any kind of esophageal atresia repair for Type C anomaly. The reported incidence of recurrent TEF is 3–14% in various series [10]. The most common causes of recurrence of fistula are early minor anastomotic leak causing inflammation in the area with exposed mucosa on the esophageal as well as tracheal side. Usually after suture trans-fixation of the TE fistula, the mucosa is everted and exposed to the adjacent anastomosis and is in persistent contact if there is no intervening tissue between the two. In the event of a leak, either minor or major mucosa on the esophageal anastomosis is also exposed, and as a natural process, it establishes a tract with the trachea with epithelization of the tract. This results in rTEF. This is accentuated if there is associated anastomotic stricture and narrowing resulting in the pooling of secretions in the upper esophagus not easily passing down in the esophagus. This process can happen any time around 2 weeks to 6 months with peak incidence around 3–4 months after primary surgery. Some authors have reported the use of clips as a causative factor and its migration exposing the fistula mucosa.

Strategies to Avoid rTEF

During primary TEF repair while ligating the fistula, the possibility of recurrence should be considered, and steps should be taken to avoid these complications. The ligation of the fistula should be done by trans-fixation, and if there is exposed mucosa abutting the anastomotic suture line, the surgeon should look to interpose some available tissue between the two. A pleural flap can be taken from the surrounding the area, and placing it between the two can help avoid a rTEF even if there is a minor leak. Gupta M et al. [11] and Simsek M et al. [12] used a free and vascularized pleural flap reinforcement of the anastomosis and reported successful outcomes. The other component of prevention is to have a wide anastomosis to avoid stricture and stenosis and preserve vascularity while mobilizing esophageal pouches. Use of clips should be avoided as far as possible, and proper suture trans-fixation should be done with nonabsorbable suture.

Treatment of rTEF

Once diagnosed to have a recurrent TEF, the condition can be approached via thoracoscopy. Several authors have demonstrated the usefulness of thoracoscopy over open repair due to the excellent magnification of the fistula area.

Endoscopic cauterization and surgical repair by open or thoracoscopy are two main alternatives for rTEF.

Endoscopic Cauterization

There are reports of the use of endoscopic cauterization of the fistulous tract from the tracheal side. Lelonge Y et al. [13] used trichloroacetic acid which is a sclerosant that causes chemical burn to the mucosa and causes obliteration by fibrosis. This requires multiple endoscopic procedures, and the authors reported 100% success in 12 patients with an average of 2 endoscopy procedures in their set of patients. This method, however, is not established, and apart from few reports, there is no proper evidence for the success of this method, and it is mostly used as individual practice.

Thoracoscopy and Surgical Division of rTEF

Thoracoscopy can be done for approaching rTEF irrespective of the first surgery being done by open or by thoracoscopy. It will be easier if the first surgery was done by thoracoscopy and there was no or minimal leak of anastomosis. Open surgery and major leak will cause adhesion, and there will be difficult trocar placement and difficult esophageal and fistula dissection. Thoracoscopy provides excellent visualization of the upper mediastinal area, and precise dissection can be done for the fistula. The esophagus is preferably looped below and above the fistula (Fig. 9.6), and the fistula can be identified either by a preplaced guidewire in the tract or by expansion of the fistula with ventilation. Once identified the fistula is ligated with nonabsorbable suture, and any available tissue (pleural tissue) is placed between the two cut ends to avoid recurrence (Video 9.1).

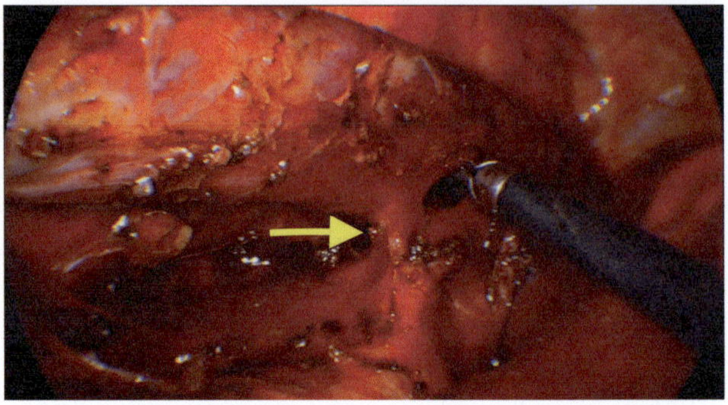

Fig. 9.6 Intraoperative view of recurrent TEF (arrow)

9.2.2.2 Anastomotic Stricture as Early Complication Within 3 Months of Surgery

Causes/Incidence

Anastomotic stricture after thoracoscopic repair is the most common complication, and the reported incidence ranges from 10% to 30% in various meta-analysis [14]. This was reported as same incidence as compared to open repair in several meta-analysis discussed in Chap. 11. Anastomotic stricture is one of the earliest complications in short term and is dependent on the quality of anastomosis achieved during initial repair. Development of stricture is multifactorial, and these factors can be classified a direct and indirect.

Long gap atresia with anastomosis done under tension and a resolved leak in the early postoperative period are the two most direct factors indicating stricture formation in early follow-up, and these patients need to be followed closely for early dilatation. There are other indirect and less established factors which include preterm low birth weight, the presence of cardiac anomaly, and severity of gastroesophageal reflux. Of these presence and severity of gastroesophageal reflux have a very close association as reflux tends to increase the inflammation and fibrosis process in the unhealthy mucosa of the anastomosis.

How to Prevent a Stricture

Prevention of stricture begins from achieving a tension-free anastomosis at initial surgery. This may not be possible every time due to gap issues and in cases with higher gap tension will be inevitable. Management of long-gap esophageal atresia and techniques to achieve primary anastomosis with least possible tension are discussed in detail in Chap. 11. The other strategy is to preempt the stricture with early dilatation in follow-up in high-risk patients. So, patients with adverse direct factors as mentioned above should be followed by early dye study as early as 6 weeks to know the anastomosis status and do prophylactic dilatation.

Subjective Evaluation of Stricture on Esophagogram

Contrast esophagogram obtained after esophageal anastomosis is the standard practice. Its use and timing are variable with different centers. In the author's practice timing of esophagograms will depend on leak risk probability. In patients who are classified as *high-risk*, i.e., with the anastomosis under tension and leak in the recovery period, there will be two esophagograms. The first esophagogram is done before the initiation of oral feeds after thoracoscopic repair; this is done once the leak is resolved. The authors have reported a quantitative index in the form of *esophageal anastomotic caliber index (EACI)* which correlates well with the risk of stricture formation. This is a ratio measured on X-ray images of esophagograms with diameters at, above, and below the level of anastomosis (Figs. 9.7 and 9.8). The average of D/DU and D/DL will be the EACI. If the EACI is 0.35, then this means that the anastomosis area is 35% of a normal esophagus diameter. If EACI [15] is adverse (below 0.65), the chances of stricture formation are high, and a second dye study is done after 8 weeks of discharge. If the EACI is favorable (>0.65), the dye study can be done after 3 months of discharge. If, on the second dye study, there is stricture, then serial endoscopic balloon dilatations are done for managing stricture.

For *low-risk* patients with easy anastomosis and minimal tension, they are followed clinically with a single dye study at 3 months of age. After this any repeat study required can be done to assess gastroesophageal reflux and not for stricture.

Redo Thoracoscopy and Revision of Anastomosis with Stricture

For established stricture with failed endoscopic dilatation, the management includes revision of anastomosis. Thoracoscopy is a viable alternative in these patients. Figure 9.9 shows the presence of stricture after a thoracoscopic repair, and this was revised by redo thoracoscopy thus avoiding thoracotomy again. Thoracoscopy is also an alternative for stricture repair even after a previous open esophageal atresia repair. However, the presence of lung adhesions is more in this instance.

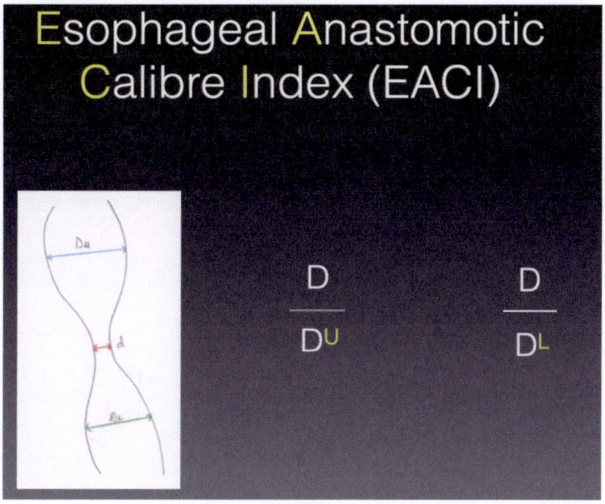

Fig. 9.7 Ratios and calculation used for estimating esophageal anastomotic caliber index

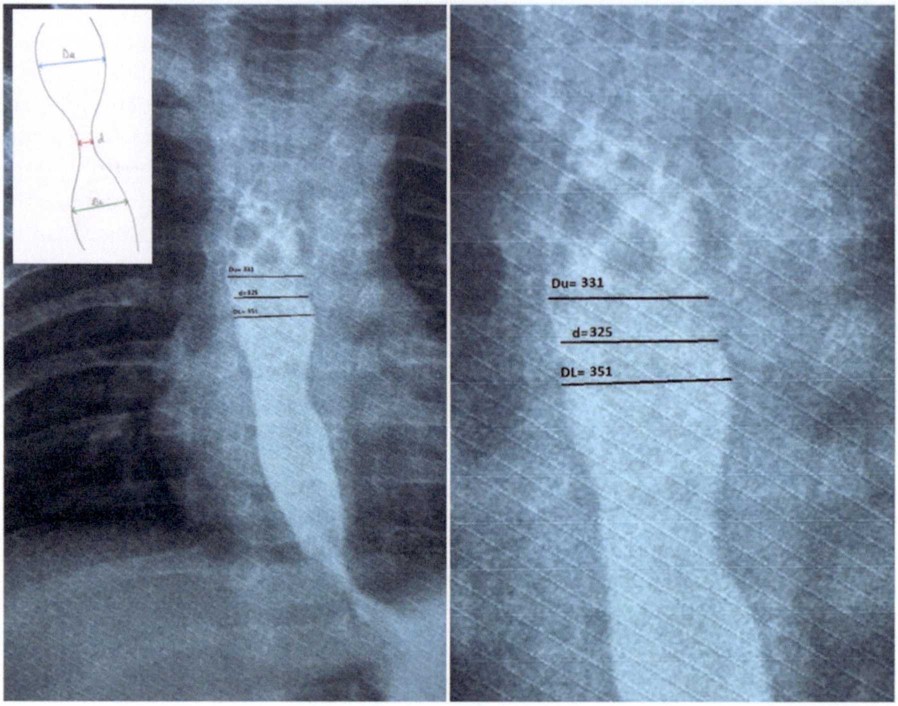

Fig. 9.8 Measurements for EACI calculation done on contrast esophagogram X-ray films

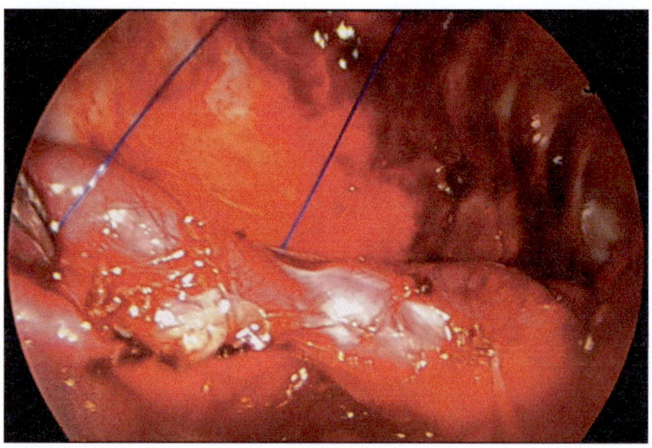

Fig. 9.9 Intraoperative thoracoscopic view showing stricture at the previous anastomosis site. This was revised by thoracoscopic excision of stricture area and revision of anastomosis

Godoy J et al. [1] reported a series of four patients who underwent thoracoscopic reentry into the chest after an early leak. The leak site was re-sutured with Polydiaxone suture and had successful outcome with resolution of leak. This approach is different to conventional norms where after an unresolving leak, the main treatment is diversion (Video 9.2).

9.3 Conclusions

To conclude on the discussion in this chapter, anastomotic leak and air leak after surgery are common, and multiple factors exist to decide on the management. Chylothorax is a rare but serious complication after esophageal repair, and the anatomy of the thoracic duct should always be in surgeons mind while dissecting the esophageal pouches. Both the surgical management and conservative management of this condition are very difficult with high mortality rate. The indications of diversion should be in accordance with the risk stratification of the esophageal anastomosis, and decision-making should be guided by the gap and tension during initial repair. Re-suturing of the esophagus is a viable alternative. Newer approaches of redo thoracoscopy have been reported and help in saving repeat thoracotomy and native esophagus by avoiding diversion.

Re-fistulation and stricture are common in early follow-up and can be managed in several ways. Repeat thoracoscopy is an option in these patients who were otherwise subjected to thoracotomy.

References

1. Godoy J, Ferraris T, Guelfand M. Early management of esophageal leak in esophageal atresia: changing paradigms. J Laparoendosc Adv Surg Tech A. 2020;30(8):923–6.
2. van Lennep M, Singendonk MMJ, Dall'Oglio L, Gottrand F, Krishnan U, Terheggen-Lagro SWJ, et al. Oesophageal atresia. Nat Rev Dis Primers. 2019;5(1):26.
3. Huang JX, Hong SM, Chen Q, Wang ZC, Wu DM, Hong JJ, et al. Risk factors for anastomotic complications after one-stage anastomosis for oesophageal atresia. J Cardiothorac Surg. 2021;16(1):176.
4. Seleim HM, Wishahy AMK, Magdy B, Elseoudi M, Zakaria RH, Kaddah SN, et al. The dilemma after an unforeseen aortic arch anomalies at thoracoscopic repair of esophageal atresia: is curtailing surgery still a necessity? Scand J Surg. 2022;111(2):14574969221090487.
5. Lal DR, Gadepalli SK, Downard CD, Minneci PC, Knezevich M, Chelius TH, et al. Infants with esophageal atresia and right aortic arch: characteristics and outcomes from the Midwest Pediatric Surgery Consortium. J Pediatr Surg. 2019;54(4):688–92.
6. Zhao J, Yang S, Li S, Wang P, Zhang Y, Zhao Y, et al. Retrospective analysis of pneumothorax after repair of esophageal atresia/tracheoesophageal fistula. BMC Pediatr. 2021;21(1):543.
7. Besendorfer M, Muller H, Weiss C, Wagner A, Schellerer V, Hoerning A, et al. Association of clinical factors with postoperative complications of esophageal atresia. Pediatr Neonatol. 2021;62(1):55–63.

8. Karabulut R, Turkyilmaz Z, Kaya C, Sonmez K. A brief comment on pneumothorax during extubation period of esophageal atresia repair. Pediatr Neonatol. 2021;62(2):231.
9. Shirotsuki R, Uchida H, Tanaka Y, Shirota C, Yokota K, Murase N, et al. Novel thoracoscopic navigation surgery for neonatal chylothorax using indocyanine-green fluorescent lymphography. J Pediatr Surg. 2018;53(6):1246–9.
10. Wang J, Zhang M, Pan W, Wu W, Yan W, Cai W. Management of recurrent tracheoesophageal fistula after esophageal atresia and follow-up. Dis Esophagus. 2017;30(9):1–8.
11. Gupta M, Mahajan JK, Bawa M, Rao KL. Esophageal atresia and tracheoesophageal fistula: effect of pleural cover on anastomotic dehiscence. J Indian Assoc Pediatr Surg. 2011;16(2):50–3.
12. Simsek M, Mert M. A new approach to tense end-to-end anostomosis in primary surgical repair of esophageal atresia: vascularized pleural flap. Chirurgia. 2021;116(1):60–5.
13. Lelonge Y, Varlet F, Varela P, Saitua F, Fourcade L, Gutierrez R, et al. Chemocauterization with trichloroacetic acid in congenital and recurrent tracheoesophageal fistula: a minimally invasive treatment. Surg Endosc. 2016;30(4):1662–6.
14. Iacona RV, Saxena AK. Thoracoscopic repair of esophageal atresia with distal tracheoesophageal fistula (type C): systematic review. Surg Laparosc Endosc Percutan Tech. 2020;30(4):388–93.
15. Kumar R, Kanojia RP, Gupta PK. Esophageal anastomotic caliber index: assessment tool for measuring outcome after thoracoscopic and open repair of esophageal atresia with tracheaesophageal fistula. J Ped Endosc Surg. 2021;3:123–7.

Long-Gap Esophageal Atresia and Thoracoscopic Approach

10

Contents

Learning Objectives
1. Growth potential of esophageal pouches
2. Thoracoscopic management options for pure esophageal atresia
3. Thoracoscopic management options for Type C esophageal atresia
4. Algorithm for management
5. Current evidence

10.1 Introduction

Long-gap esophageal atresia with or without fistula is not so uncommon. Lewis Spitz [1] in 2007 reported the incidence of EA-TEF as 86%, with isolated atresia without fistula being 7% and 4% as H-type TEF of all patients. Approximately 7% of esophageal atresias are long gap where the primary anastomosis is not possible, and a staged procedure is required. The conventional treatment for long-gap EA-TEF is fistula ligation, diversion, and later esophageal replacement. For esophageal

R. P. Kanojia, *Thoracoscopic Repair of Esophageal Atresia*,
https://doi.org/10.1007/978-981-97-5695-7_10

atresia without fistula, diversion and later esophageal replacement are done with stomach or colonic conduit. In either case, the native esophagus is lost, and so are the natural functions of the esophagus. The replacement gut serves as a passive conduit with many complications in long term. Several studies in the past have established the growth potential of upper and lower pouches with the stimulus of traction. With this fact in mind, surgeons have always strived to save the native esophagus in some form or another. In the past five decades with open surgery, many reports of successful elongation of the upper pouch have been documented by various traction techniques [2]. However, traction often required repeated thoracotomies to do the staged procedure. This contributed to morbidity and mortality, especially in centers where the level of neonatal care is suboptimal. With the advent of thoracoscopy, requirement of morbid thoracotomy in the fragile newborn was eliminated. The current chapter discusses the procedures that utilize thoracoscopy as a staged approach for long-gap esophageal atresia. The recent evidence in the literature for these procedures is also discussed.

10.2 Growth Potential of Atretic Esophagus with Traction (the Basic Premise of the Concept)

The esophagus is a dynamically growing organ. The growth rate is significant in the first few weeks of life. In patients of esophageal atresia, the two atretic ends, the upper pouch and lower pouch, have the potential to grow both in length and diameter. This is similar to other parts of the gut. This is established by the fact that in most of the cases, the upper pouch is more developed than the lower pouch because in utero fetus has been swallowing amniotic fluid which provides the hydro-distention stimulus for the upper pouch growth. Similar stimulus is not available to the lower pouch, and hence, it is always thin and hypoplastic. Similarly, in pure atresia patients, the lower pouch and the stomach never get this distention stimulus, and hence, the lower esophagus stump and gastric capacity are always small in pure esophageal atresia patients. Distention and hydro-stretch as stimulus for growth are well-established phenomenon in human physiology and growth of organs [3]. Urinary bladder in patients with bilateral ectopic ureter is always hypoplastic as it never accumulates urine and distends in untreated patients. Similarly, exstrophy bladder patients always have small, underdeveloped bladder plates as they have never had the stimulus of distention and growth. However, once the bladder is closed at birth and with enough resistance at the bladder neck, they grow with a reasonable rate with the growth of child and hydro-distention. Another example of lack of volume growth in the absence of distention is in patients with gastroschisis who will have small capacity abdominal cavity with all the bowel outside the abdomen.

Researchers have always pondered over the pathophysiological basis of axial traction as stimulus for the growth of the esophagus. Krystian Toczewski et al. established in vitro experimental model that axial traction leads to a gain in length in the duck esophagus [4]. He also established that intermittent traction is better than continuous traction. Similarly, Christina Oetzmann et al. [5] had similar observation with the porcine esophagus. Both the authors also deliberated on the biomechanics of the esophagus under traction with no clear physiological explanation. The first author concluded that traction in the direction of growth provided maximum gain in length.

10.3 Long-Gap Pure Esophageal Atresia

Pure esophageal atresia is universally long gap with the absence of fistula in the lower pouch (Fig. 10.1). The gap distance in this category of patients is sometimes up to six vertebral bodies. This gap length is impossible to bridge primarily. Ten percent of these patients may have an upper pouch fistula [6]. The conventional approach for the esophagus-preserving surgery was first described by Foker and Kimura. Foker described the method of intrathoracic esophageal elongation, ultimately achieving enough length to make primary anastomosis [7]. Similarly, Kimura achieved the same method by serial extrathoracic elongation by moving cervical esophagostomy caudally in a stepwise manner [8]. Both are staged and open procedures and require multiple thoracotomies in neonate which may not be tolerated by all patients especially in low resource settings. Foker [7] himself

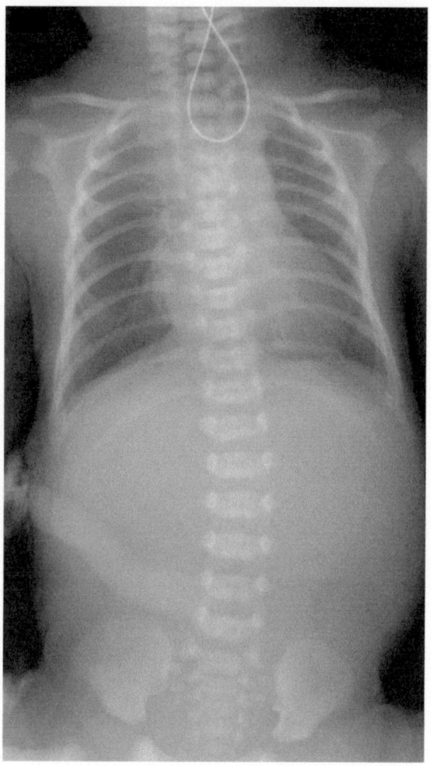

Fig. 10.1 X-ray showing high upper pouch in long-gap esophageal atresia. The gap is approximately 5–6 vertebra long

acknowledged that it will be of tremendous advantage to the baby, if the serial lengthening can be done without thoracotomy using minimal invasive technique.

10.3.1 Technique

At the initial diagnosis of long-gap pure esophageal atresia without fistula, the general practice is to first establish a feeding portal by gastrostomy. This can be done by either open procedure or by laparoscopy. Tube gastrostomy serves many purposes apart from feeding. The volume distention done during feeding helps the stomach grow in capacity and this later gives the option of a gastric tube conduit if at all esophageal replacement is inevitable. The gastrostomy also fixes the stomach to the abdomen and provides a counter traction to the traction which will be applied to the lower esophageal pouch and prevents the cardia of stomach travelling up into thorax during the esophageal elongation procedure.

Bronchoscopy can also be done at the start of this procedure to rule out an upper pouch fistula. At this stage cervical esophagostomy is not done, and in the same sitting or when the patient is stable, thoracoscopy is done to set up the internal traction elongation. The patient is positioned in the same position as in thoracoscopy for Type C atresia. Similarly, ports, position, and access are also the same. The proximal esophagus is mobilized first which is high up in the thoracic inlet. If a proximal pouch fistula is present, then it is dealt with at this stage. The pouch is circumferentially mobilized by careful dissection. Every attempt is made to be as nontraumatic as possible to the wall of the upper pouch. Minor trauma, tears, or crushing forces to the wall of the upper pouch will lead to inflammatory adhesions to the chest wall and the lungs. This will make the subsequent stages of pouch mobilization difficult. Once mobilization is complete, the lower pouch is searched for and is mobilized. The lower pouch in general is thin and hypoplastic and has poor vascularity. The pouch is grasped by atraumatic graspers or lifted by stay sutures. The mobilization should be up to the esophageal hiatus. With enough mobilization, the fundus of the stomach will be visible in the thoracoscopic view. This is the reason that all these patients require fundoplication later. Once mobilization is complete, the traction sutures are taken through the upper and lower pouches. The sutures are taken in a way in the upper pouch so that the mucosa is included in the bite. This is achieved by keeping a stiff size 10 Fr. feeding tube in the upper pouch through the mouth. If the bites are taken without the mucosa, there may be lag in the growth of the muscularis layer and the mucosa, leading to tension in the anastomosis with poor wall strength at the time of primary anastomosis. Pledgets can be used to prevent suture biting off from esophageal tissue. The sutures are then crossed out and retrieved out of the chest wall through intercostal space (Fig. 10.2). The threads are secured on small artery forceps. A clip is applied to the tip of the lower and upper pouch so that the distance between the two can be assessed on X-rays. There are options on where to keep the traction sutures. Patkwoski D et al. [9] demonstrated that the traction sutures are brought out of the chest wall as long threads and the tension can be modified under fluoroscopy or bedside to facilitate elongation. Some other authors

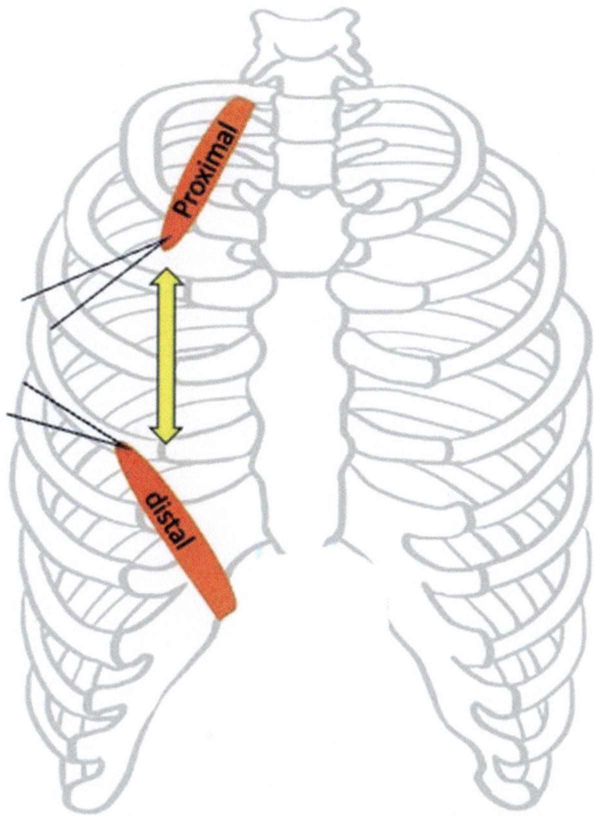

Fig. 10.2 Schematic diagram showing traction sutures applied to the upper and lower pouch for elongation

tied the traction sutures internally to the ribs or looped it around the rib before tying it internally [10]. The choice of suture material is variable. Non-absorbable monofilament sutures are preferred; however, 5/0 ethibond has been used in majority of the reports. The baby returns to the intensive care and is sedated and ventilated. In general, 2–3 days of traction time is given. Everyday morning serial chest radiographs are done to assess the gap by measuring the distance between the clips. It is not advisable to prolong the traction time for more than 3 days as adhesions will be forming between the pouches and the endothoracic fascia and the lung tissue, making subsequent stage more difficult. After 3 days no matter what the distance is achieved, the thoracoscopy is repeated. Same port sites can be utilized, and gentle release of adhesions is done. The gap is assessed again for the feasibility of safe primary anastomosis with acceptable tension. If this is possible, then anastomosis is completed. If not, then the traction sutures are reapplied, and this time can exit through a higher space for more efficient traction. In general, after two stages majority of the pouches will come close enough for primary anastomosis.

There are several avenues of failure with this approach. The most common is the biting of the sutures and failure of the applied traction. This is managed by reapplying of the sutures at a subsequent stage. The other problem is the failure of the

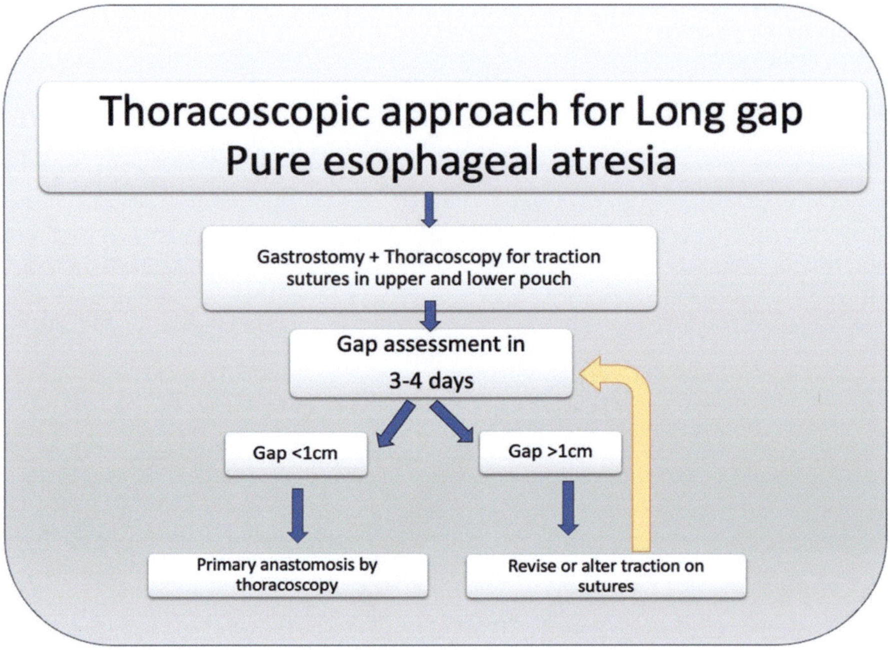

Fig. 10.3 Algorithm for thoracoscopic approach for long-gap pure esophageal atresia

growth of the pouch even with 4–6 days of traction. This is usually common in preterm small for gestational age babies, and they will need diversion with replacement later.

The traction duration is important to understand. Majority of esophageal pouches will grow long enough over a period of 4–6 days with one intervention. If gap is not reduced by this time, it becomes unlikely that it will reduce further by more days of traction. The maximum number of days mentioned in the longest series of 10 patients with this procedure is 10 days. Figure 10.3 shows the management algorithm for long-gap pure esophageal atresia.

10.4 Long-Gap Esophageal Atresia with Fistula

The long-gap Type C atresia is relatively easier to deal with as the gap length to cover is mostly 3–4 vertebral length (Fig. 10.4). Type C requires fistula ligation as a priority, and thoracoscopy is done as the first procedure. With gentle dissection only fistula ligation is done. A clip or suture obliteration with no disconnection with the trachea is done. At this stage the surgeon can opt to place internal traction sutures in upper pouch as done in the long-gap atresia. Other alternative is to leave the upper

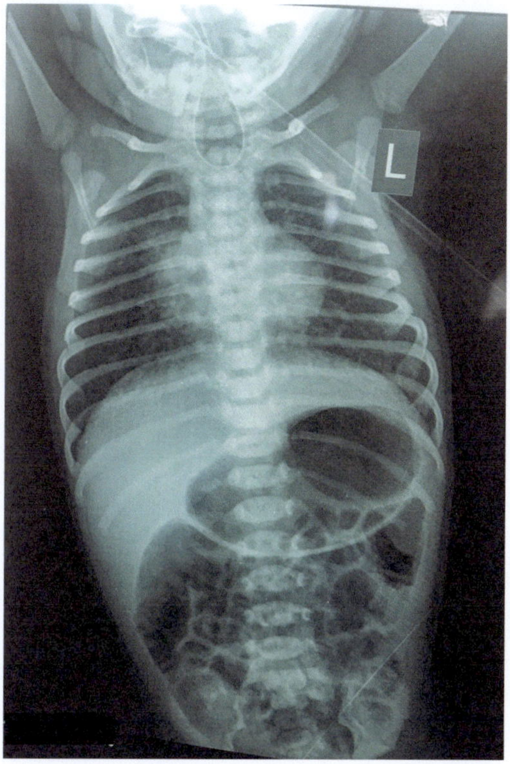

Fig. 10.4 Chest X-ray for Type C esophageal atresia with tracheoesophageal fistula. Note the high location of upper pouch indicating a gap of three to four vertebrae

pouch untouched, and a replogle suction is placed. In postoperative period repeated bouginage is done daily as bedside procedure with the expectation of pouch elongation and growth. This may require a few days to a couple of weeks of and will require active replogle suction round the clock to prevent aspiration pneumonia. Once the radiographs show the gap is short enough for anastomosis, thoracoscopy is done to perform anastomosis. Suna Sun et al. [11] reported 12 infants with bouginage followed by esophageal anastomosis. This is discussed in detail in the following segments.

Figure 10.5 shows the management algorithm for long-gap Type C esophageal atresia.

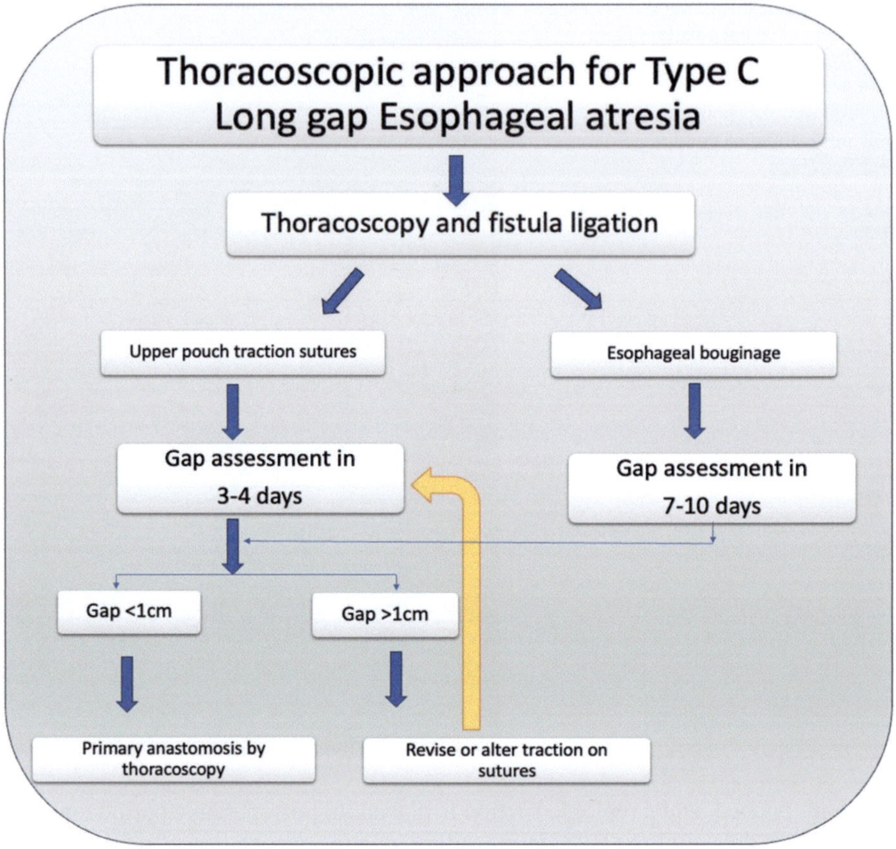

Fig. 10.5 Algorithm for thoracoscopic approach for long gap Type C esophageal atresia with tracheoesophageal fistula

10.5 Results from Literature

There is paucity of sufficient data on the thoracoscopic staged approach for long-gap atresia. The largest series is reported by *David Vander Ze*, who reported ten patients in 2015 [12]. He reported failure in two patients with failure of elongation and successful staged anastomosis in eight patients. He initially used gastrostomy in these patients which was later converted to gastropexy. The mean weight of patients was 2.3 kg. Four patients had a proximal fistula. Two of these fistulas were approached via the neck, and in remaining two were ligated during thoracoscopic mobilization. These ten patients required a mean of three to four procedures in achieving the primary anastomosis. Table 10.1 provides a summary of cases reported for long-gap esophageal atresia treated with thoracoscopic approach.

Zhenis Sakuov et al. [9] reported as series of three patients. These were done during a surgical demonstration with Dr. Patkowski. Two patients had upper pouch

Table 10.1 Summary of cases reported for long-gap esophageal atresia treated with thoracoscopic approach

Year of study	Authors	Number of patients	Remarks
2022	Zhenis Sakuov et al. [9]	3	First report from Kzakhstan, successful with three patients one needed dilatation
2021	Satoshi Ieiri et al. [14]	1	Five vertebrae gap, anastomosed after 5 weeks
2018	Suna Sun et al. [11]	7/12	Pouch bouginage was done as a bedside procedure
2018	Bartosz Bogusz et al. [10]	4	Age at anastomosis was 11, 10, and 9 days and 3.5 months
2017	Takahisa Tainaka et al. [15]	5	Minor anastomotic leak in 2 patients.
2015	David C. van der Zee et al. [12]	10	Failure in two patients with failure of elongation and successful staged anastomosis in eight patients
2013	Yujiro Tanaka et al. [13]	1	Used complete internal traction with ribs
2013	Go Miyano et al. [16]	1	Used Kimura's extrathoracic elongation with a thoracoscopic anastomosis once adequate length was achieved
2011	David C. van der Zee et al. [17]	4	This is the first series of staged thoracoscopic traction and anastomosis
2007	David C. van der Zee et al. [18]	1	First report for internal traction and anastomosis

fistula. Traction sutures were applied in all three patients thoracoscopically. To complete the esophageal anastomosis, two of the three patients needed only one traction procedure, and the third patient needed two traction procedures. The average days to complete esophageal anastomosis was 2–4 days. There was no anastomotic leakage in these three patients. Esophageal stenosis was present in one patient in follow-up treated by dilatation. The follow-up duration of these patients was 10–13 months.

Yujiro Tanaka et al. [13] reported a 2300 gm neonate with pure esophageal atresia. As a first-stage procedure, he did a gastrostomy and a thoracoscopic mobilization of proximal and distal esophagus. He was able to bridge a gap of six vertebrae to one by applying internal traction sutures which were tied internally to ribs. Esophageal anastomosis was done on day 26 of life. Seven-month follow-up duration was reported. He concluded that the use of internal traction sutures has less chance for infection as compared to the external traction sutures.

Suna Sun et al. [11] reported a series of 12 patients where esophageal bouginage was done as a primary method of upper and lower pouch esophageal lengthening. Later they did primary esophageal anastomosis by thoracoscopy in seven patients and by thoracotomy in five patients. All patients received a gastrostomy. The pouch bouginage is done as a bedside procedure. The mean duration for these patients was 7.4 weeks.

Table 10.1 summarizes the series and case reports reported in the literature. A total of 37 patients are documented with a success rate of nearly 100% with no mortality.

10.6 Conclusions

To conclude, the preservation of the native esophagus is of high priority in esophageal atresia. This can be achieved by the newer methods of staged traction and elongation as described in this chapter. The traction techniques are feasible and have been successful in achieving primary anastomosis. Anastomotic leak, stricture, and severe reflux are the tradeoff morbidity which happens with this approach. Considering the morbidity of esophageal replacement, these tradeoffs are acceptable and give better quality of life when compared to esophageal replacement procedures. Thoracoscopy offers the advantage of avoiding repeated thoracotomies. The literature has limited evidence as there are very few patients, surgeons, and centers who have undergone and done these procedures successfully.

References

1. Spitz L. Oesophageal atresia. Orphanet J Rare Dis. 2007;2:24.
2. von Allmen D, Wijnen RM. Bridging the gap in the repair of long-gap esophageal atresia: still questions on diagnostics and treatment. Eur J Pediatr Surg. 2015;25(4):312–7.
3. Chai TC, Zhang CO, Shoenfelt JL, Johnson HW Jr, Warren JW, Keay S. Bladder stretch alters urinary heparin-binding epidermal growth factor and antiproliferative factor in patients with interstitial cystitis. J Urol. 2000;163(5):1440–4.
4. Toczewski K, Gerus S, Kaczorowski M, Kozun M, Wolicka J, Bobrek K, et al. Biomechanics of esophageal elongation with traction sutures on experimental animal model. Sci Rep. 2022;12(1):3420.
5. Oetzmann von Sochaczewski C, Tagkalos E, Lindner A, Lang H, Heimann A, Schroder A, et al. Esophageal biomechanics revisited: a tale of tenacity, anastomoses, and suture bite lengths in swine. Ann Thorac Surg. 2019;107(6):1670–7.
6. Long AM, Tyraskis A, Allin B, Burge DM, Knight M. Oesophageal atresia with no distal tracheoesophageal fistula: management and outcomes from a population-based cohort. J Pediatr Surg. 2017;52(2):226–30.
7. Foker JE, Kendall Krosch TC, Catton K, Munro F, Khan KM. Long-gap esophageal atresia treated by growth induction: the biological potential and early follow-up results. Semin Pediatr Surg. 2009;18(1):23–9.
8. Kimura K, Nishijima E, Tsugawa C, Collins DL, Lazar EL, Stylianos S, et al. Multistaged extrathoracic esophageal elongation procedure for long gap esophageal atresia: experience with 12 patients. J Pediatr Surg. 2001;36(11):1725–7.
9. Sakuov Z, Dzhenalaev D, Ospanov M, Rustemov D, Lozovoy V, Erekeshov A, et al. Long-gap esophageal atresia repair using staged thoracoscopic internal traction: the first Kazakhstan experience. J Laparoendosc Adv Surg Tech A. 2022;32(12):1265–8.
10. Bogusz B, Patkowski D, Gerus S, Rasiewicz M, Gorecki W. Staged thoracoscopic repair of Long-gap esophageal atresia without temporary gastrostomy. J Laparoendosc Adv Surg Tech A. 2018;28(12):1510–2.

11. Sun S, Pan W, Wu W, Gong Y, Shi J, Wang J. Elongation of esophageal segments by bougienage stretching technique for long gap esophageal atresia to achieve delayed primary anastomosis by thoracotomy or thoracoscopic repair: a first experience from China. J Pediatr Surg. 2018;53(8):1584–7.
12. van der Zee DC, Gallo G, Tytgat SH. Thoracoscopic traction technique in long gap esophageal atresia: entering a new era. Surg Endosc. 2015;29(11):3324–30.
13. Tanaka Y, Uchida H, Kawashima H, Sato K, Takazawa S, Jimbo T, et al. Successful two-stage thoracoscopic repair of long-gap esophageal atresia using simple internal traction and delayed primary anastomosis in a neonate: report of a case. Surg Today. 2013;43(8):906–9.
14. Ieiri S, Kai H, Hirose R. Thoracoscopic intraoperative esophageal close technique for long-gap esophageal atresia. Asian J Endosc Surg. 2022;15(1):240–3.
15. Tainaka T, Uchida H, Tanano A, Shirota C, Hinoki A, Murase N, et al. Two-stage thoracoscopic repair of long-gap esophageal atresia using internal traction is safe and feasible. J Laparoendosc Adv Surg Tech A. 2017;27(1):71–5.
16. Miyano G, Okuyama H, Koga H, Okawada M, Doi T, Takahashi T, et al. Type-A long-gap esophageal atresia treated by thoracoscopic esophagoesophagostomy after sequential extrathoracic esophageal elongation (Kimura's technique). Pediatr Surg Int. 2013;29(11):1171–5.
17. van der Zee DC. Thoracoscopic elongation of the esophagus in long-gap esophageal atresia. J Pediatr Gastroenterol Nutr. 2011;52(Suppl 1):S13–S5.
18. van der Zee DC, Vieirra-Travassos D, Kramer WL, Tytgat SH. Thoracoscopic elongation of the esophagus in long gap esophageal atresia. J Pediatr Surg. 2007;42(10):1785–8.

Thoracoscopic Versus Open Repair for Esophageal Atresia: The Current Evidence

11

Contents

Learning Objectives

1. Literature review of series reporting comparison between open and thoracoscopic repair of esophageal atresia

11.1 Introduction

Open thoracotomy repair for esophageal atresia has been practiced for the last 100 years and is a gold-standard procedure for the correction of esophageal atresia. With the continued evolution of surgical techniques and the development of minimal access techniques, pediatric surgeons have pushed the limits with neonatal minimal access procedures like congenital diaphragmatic hernia and TREAT. This has paralleled the development of neonatal anesthesia and intensive care. Thoracoscopic repair of esophageal atresia was first reported in 1999 [1], and since then for the last two and a half decades, the procedure has been adopted by surgeons worldwide with increasing success percentage. With every new adoption, there are always questions about the comparison with the established practice and gold standard. Several large series comparing outcomes are now available for both open and thoracoscopic repair of esophageal atresia.

R. P. Kanojia, *Thoracoscopic Repair of Esophageal Atresia*,
https://doi.org/10.1007/978-981-97-5695-7_11

When PubMed is searched for thoracoscopic repair for esophageal atresia, close to 100 papers are published. These are a standalone cohort study that is either deliberating on various aspects of the operation or is being compared with open repair.

This chapter aims to summarize the current literature available on the two methods (open and thoracoscopic) and presents the evidence available. We do not aim to deliberate if one is superior to the other.

11.2 Review of Systematic Reviews and Meta-Analysis

The two methods have been compared over several parameters, and to date there is no double-blind randomized controlled trial (RCT) to show if one is better than the other.

We searched the literature exclusively for systematic reviews and meta-analyses which analyzed series comparing outcomes between open repair and TREAT. The search duration was fixed between 1999 and 2023 which is the period of existence of TREAT. Table 11.1 summarizes the six systematic reviews retrieved by the above search criteria (searched in Jan 2024).

Falharty E et al. [2] is the recent most systematic review and meta-analysis with 14 studies included in the analysis. There is aggregated patient data for 355 TREAT and 1077 open repair patients. This series had many common data points of analysis with the other three meta-analyses. Anastomotic leak rate was 14.3% and 12.4%. Stricture was 27.7% and 25.3% mean duration of surgery was 170.8 and 148.4 min in TREAT and the open group, respectively. Mean length of hospital stay (LOS) was 31 and 41 days for TREAT and the open group. There were some other parameters which were analyzed and were not considered in earlier studies. They reported major comorbidities in 60% and 66.8% of patients with TREAT and the open group. The mortality was 2.6% and 2.8% in the two groups, respectively. Redo surgery was required in 6.8% of TREAT procedures and 7.8% of open repairs. All these differences were not found to be statistically significant except for the data on major comorbidities.

Table 11.1 Systematic review and meta-analysis reported in literature

Sr no.	Year of publication	Authors	Number of articles included	Totals no of patients analyzed
1.	2023	Flaherty E et al. [2]	14	1432 (355 TREAT and 1077 open repair)
2.	2021	Gustaf Drevin [3]	17	1043 patients, 695 open repair and 348 thoracoscopic repair
3.	2019	Colin Way [4]	14	Meta-analysis using a Delphi questionnaire method
4.	2017	Chun Wu [5]	10	447
5.	2016	Yang Y et al. [6]	8	452
6.	2012	Francesca AB et al. [7]	4	69 + 97 = 166

They finally concluded that the benefits of avoiding thoracotomy with TREAT is a major advantage, and patients have less pain and better visualization, and the two procedures are very much comparable.

Gustaf Drevin et al. [3] did a systematic review and meta-analysis with 17 studies including 1043 patients (695 open repair and 348 thoracoscopic repair). He reported shorter hospital stay with thoracoscopy. There was shorter time to oral feed with fewer musculoskeletal complications. The leak rate was also less as compared to open. Like other studies he also reported longer operative time in thoracoscopy.

Colin Way et al. [4] did a systematic review and meta-analysis using a Delphi questionnaire method. There were 14 studies included. He found no statistical difference in primary outcome of esophageal atresia with thoracoscopic or open approach. There was no difference in the leak rate (odds ratio 1.55), esophageal stricture (odds ratio 1.92), and need for fundoplication (odds ratio 1.22). However, operative time was more in thoracoscopy group than in the open group. He concluded that TREAT is safe and there is no increased morbidity when compared to open approach.

Chun Wu et al. [5] did a systematic review and meta-analysis for clinical outcomes between TREAT and open repair in 2017. This study included 447 patients (51% TREAT and 49% open repair) in ten studies. More additional parameters were studied in this analysis, and they reported similar outcomes as seen in the previous three analysis. The occurrence of leak was studied in eight articles, and TREAT group did not have more occurrence of leak than open repair with odds ratio of 1.7. The rate of strictures was also similar between the two groups with odds ratio of 0.937. Postoperative ventilation time was analyzed in six studies. The authors concluded that open repair does not significantly increase the duration of postoperative ventilation. Time to first oral feed was analyzed in three studies and was similar in two groups. Length of hospital stay (LOS) was reported in three studies and said that the LOS was significantly more in the open repair; this is same as detailed above in the meta-analysis done by Yang Y et al. [6]. Same data was reported for operative time and blood loss.

He did some additional parameter assessment like fundoplication rate and gastrointestinal reflux disease (GERD) in follow-up. This data was available in three studies and reported that TREAT does not increase the requirement of postoperative GERD or requirement of fundoplication with odds ratio of 1.6. Occurrence of pulmonary complications was reported in four studies and reported that open repair does not increase the occurrence of postoperative complications with odds ratio of 1.08.

Conversion rate was reported in five studies included this meta-analysis which is not analyzed in any other meta-analysis. The rates were 4.8%, 12.5%, 11.1%, 32%, and 20% with a mean of 16% of overall conversion rate.

Yang Y et al. [6] reported a meta-analysis with eight studies published till 2016. This included 452 patients. The study reported comparative outcome on various parameters. There was no significant difference between the postoperative leaks. There were 21 leaks in 203 patients in TREAT and 18 leaks out of 216 patients with odds ratio of 1.57 in 7 studies. Six studies reported on postoperative occurrence of strictures. There were 16 strictures in 167 patients in TREAT and 26 out of 169 in open repair. This was statistically not significant with odds ratio of 0.9. Six studies reported operative time outcome comparison. Here the TREAT group has a significant longer operative time than open repair avg. 172 min versus 153 min.

Three studies reported data on time to extubation, and all three reported longer time to extubation in open repair. Mean time to extubation in thoracoscopy was 3.8 days and in open repair was 7.2 days. Odds ratio was not estimated as there was significant heterogeneity between the studies.

Only two studies in meta-analysis reported time to first oral feeding. In the thoracoscopy group this was 8.3 days, whereas in the open repair group, this was 10.9.

Five studies reported the length of hospital stay for the two groups; however, only two studies had enough data for meta-analysis which showed a mean hospital stay of 37.95 days for TREAT and 44.65 days for the open group.

This meta-analysis finally concluded that TREAT is comparable to open repair in terms of leaks and strictures.

Francesca AB et al. [7] conducted a literature review and meta-analysis for studies published till 2012. The study included four series comparing open repair with TREAT. A total of 166 patients were analyzed (69 TREAT and 97 open repair). The data point studies were anastomotic stricture, leak rate, and mean operating time. They remarked that the overall complication rate was slightly higher for all intraoperative complications in the TREAT group although this was not statistically significant (odds ratio 1.29). There was no statistically significant difference for leak rate and anastomotic stricture between the two techniques. The total leak rates for TREAT versus open repair were 8.7% and 9.3%, respectively. Similarly, the stricture rates were 8.7% and 21.7%, respectively. This seems to be high for open repair but was reported as statistically not significant. The mean operating time was comparable between the two methods: 147 min ± 20 for TREAT and 136 ± 31 for open repair. The meta-analysis concluded that TREAT provides a similar experience and outcome as compared to open repair.

11.3 Drawbacks of the Studies Analyzed

All the studies included in the above six analyses were retrospective studies. Of all the series included in this meta-analysis, there was only one RCT, and the rest were all comparative retrospective studies. The grade assessment for the studies was low to moderate and was rated as Grade C on the grading of recommendation and levels of evidence. A larger multicenter RCT is required with a long term follow-up to establish the data points highlighted by the above systematic reviews.

11.4 Conclusions

To conclude, in the past two and a half decades, the thoracoscopic approach has significantly evolved. With better instrumentation and better neonatal care, centers across the world are reporting large series. Open repair is still the gold standard and the conventional way. There is a significant amount of learning curve, and as more and more centers and surgeons are being taught thoracoscopic repair, the results are bound to get better over time. Even in the current scenario, the two procedures are comparable, and TREAT has not shown any increased incidence of complications in short or long term over open repair. In near future TREAT will become the standard of care for treating esophageal atresia neonates.

References

1. Lobe TE, Rothenberg S, Waldschmidt J, Stroedter L. Thoracoscopic repair of esophageal atresia in an infant: a surgical first. Pediatr Endosurg Innov Tech. 1999;3(3):141–8.
2. Flaherty E, Folaranmi SE. Thoracoscopic Versus Open Repair of Esophageal Atresia: A Systematic Review of Surgical Outcomes. J Laparoendosc Adv Surg Tech A. 2023;33(11):1114–20.
3. Drevin G, Andersson B, Svensson JF. Thoracoscopy or thoracotomy for esophageal atresia: a systematic review and meta-analysis. Ann Surg. 2021;274(6):945–53.
4. Way C, Wayne C, Grandpierre V, Harrison BJ, Travis N, Nasr A. Thoracoscopy vs. thoracotomy for the repair of esophageal atresia and tracheoesophageal fistula: a systematic review and meta-analysis. Pediatr Surg Int. 2019;35(11):1167–84.
5. Wu Y, Kuang H, Lv T, Wu C. Comparison of clinical outcomes between open and thoracoscopic repair for esophageal atresia with tracheoesophageal fistula: a systematic review and meta-analysis. Pediatr Surg Int. 2017;33(11):1147–57.
6. Yang YF, Dong R, Zheng C, Jin Z, Chen G, Huang YL, et al. Outcomes of thoracoscopy versus thoracotomy for esophageal atresia with tracheoesophageal fistula repair: a PRISMA-compliant systematic review and meta-analysis. Medicine (Baltimore). 2016;95(30):e4428.
7. Borruto FA, Impellizzeri P, Montalto AS, Antonuccio P, Santacaterina E, Scalfari G, et al. Thoracoscopy versus thoracotomy for esophageal atresia and tracheoesophageal fistula repair: review of the literature and meta-analysis. Eur J Pediatr Surg. 2012;22(6):415–9.

Simulation and Ex Vivo Training of Surgeons for Thoracoscopic Repair of Esophageal Atresia

12

Contents

Learning Objectives

1. Advantages of simulation-based training
2. Types of simulation
3. Validation of simulation
4. Quantitative assessment on simulators

12.1 Introduction

Training pediatric surgeons for complex minimal-access procedures is difficult and requires sophisticated and expensive resources. Traditional apprenticeship model is the age-old methodology accepted by surgeons and is considered as the best form of training. Apprenticeship model provides real-time training and assessment for a trainee and prepares them as a surgeon. However, there are several limitations with this model. The topmost reason is the limited availability of opportunities for such

R. P. Kanojia, *Thoracoscopic Repair of Esophageal Atresia*,
https://doi.org/10.1007/978-981-97-5695-7_12

training. The second problem is with centers with low volume where neonatal surgical opportunities [1] are scant and training for quaternary level procedures like thoracoscopic repair for esophageal atresia will be near to impossible. Incidence of esophageal atresia at apex centers in developed nations can be as low as 3–5 per year. Providing training with low numbers is a challenge. In the future with more and more antenatal diagnosis and interventions, these numbers for congenital anomalies are expected to go down even further.

Simulation training is the answer to these training problems, especially with neonatal surgery and esophageal atresia. Simulation training is a proven method of skill acquisition and can help the trainee to understand the anatomy, working space, and the procedure itself. More importantly simulation allows you to commit mistakes and learn from it. Learning on a live patient can raise ethical issues due to higher rates of complications. The best part of simulation is the elimination of patient complications and related ethical issues.

This chapter presents a detailed account on the forms of simulation options. It will also enumerate various training models available and their effectiveness.

12.2 Advantages of Simulation-Based Learning

The aviation industry utilizes simulation as an important tool for training. Any aviation pilot in his training journey must first go through a process of theoretical learning, simulation training, and real-time apprenticeship, before he takes over as the main pilot. There is minimum number of training hours required on the simulator to advance to the next stage. The same sequence is followed for surgical training. However, conventional system makes the surgeon jump from theoretical learning to surgical apprenticeship or even worse, to directly being the surgeon thus exposing a real-life patient to the inevitable errors of learning curve of a surgeon.

Bringing in simulation into this loop of learning has several advantages. Simulation lets you go through the same procedure repeatedly till you learn all the steps of the procedure. At the same time, it also lets you do the same procedure with possible variations because every patient is different. This prepares you better for real-life scenarios. Simulation helps you to engage in productive failure and allows you to improve on the next attempt. So effectively you are allowed to commit mistakes and learn from it. It's like crashing the plane in a flight simulator and landing it safely the next time. New age simulation models have the ability to rate the surgeons attempt based on several parameters which are discussed in forthcoming text.

12.3 Types of Simulation Based on Fidelity

There are several varieties of simulation. These can be based on the fidelity of the setup and be broadly divided into low and high fidelity. The definition of fidelity is the ability of a setup to replicate reality. Higher fidelity is closer to reality and may improve training. The simulator models described below can be classified as low and high fidelity, but in general there is no accepted clear definition of fidelity for laparoscopic simulation.

The available models can be broadly categorized as:

12.3.1 Box Endo Trainers

Deployment of box endo trainers is one of the first step toward establishing a minimal-access surgery training program. It's economical and easy to set up. The biggest advantage is that the setup can be placed anywhere ranging from home to office. The box trainers are helpful for establishing hand-eye coordination and suturing practice. The practice can be both supervised and unsupervised as there is no risk of life unlike the other models described later. The simplest of the box endo trainers provide exercises for suturing and cutting and for hand-eye coordination at a very basic level. They do not simulate the real ergonomics of an actual case. These are thus low-fidelity tools when compared to other forms of simulation. These box trainers have evolved over the last decade, and there is an increasing level of sophistication. Yousi A et al. [2] showed the use of instrument motion tracking in these endo trainers. They let the trainers perform intracorporeal suturing. The motions of hand instruments and camera were recorded using a magnetic sensing system. The motion data obtained was analyzed to assess the accuracy using summed scores by software. This eliminated the need of subjective evaluation by a supervisor and reduces the cost of the training module. These box endo trainers are nowhere close to simulating the small pediatric patient ergonomics but is a stepping stone toward the skill development. The low cost of setup makes it ideal for a center with financial constraints.

12.3.2 Cadavers and Porcine Models

The live tissue models provide the most realistic training in the field of pediatric minimal invasive surgery. It greatly enhances the ability to overcome the initial learning curve. The live animal tissue models give a real feel of the tissue and help to practice in simulated environment (Fig. 12.1). There are several reports outlining the advantages. S K Narayanan et al. [3] studied the utility of pig porcine models. This paper documented various procedures done by trainees. The procedure included esophageal anastomosis, nephrectomy, cholecystectomy, adrenalectomy, and lobectomy. This was subjectively evaluated by experts. They concluded that anesthetized animals are capable of teaching advanced minimal-access skills. The anatomy of porcine models is comparable to that of humans. It also provides training for real-time dissection of tissue and simulates actual bleeding while dissecting. This is a significant improvement from a box endo trainer which lacks such avenues. In another study Zimmermann P et al. [4] proposed the use of avian models to simulate the surgical environment. However, these were culled animals. This cuts down on the cost of anesthesia setup for the procedure. However, owing to small size of

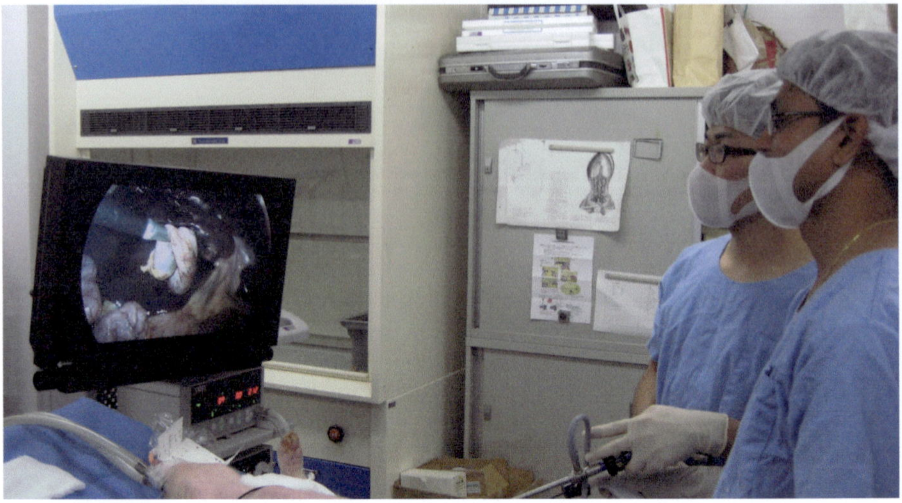

Fig. 12.1 Laparoscopic cholecystectomy being performed on live porcine animal. This gives real tissue feel and simulates a real environment for trainees

the chicken, they closely simulate the small ergonomic challenge seen in actual pediatric and neonatal procedures. The avian model setup greatly reduces the cost of procurement of the animal, and it's easily available as compared to pigs. Apart from pig and chicken, rabbit and dogs are other alternatives for live animal model simulation and have been studied by various authors for minimal-access training. Wet laboratories with animal house facilities are a must for establishing minimal-access training. This is especially useful for low-volume setup where actual patient cannot be subjected to a trainee doing the procedure.

12.3.3 Advanced Synthetic Simulators

Box endo trainers are low-fidelity and are not anatomically correct. To have high-fidelity and close to having real-life ergonomics, researchers have developed several sophisticated training models. These models comprise of a 3D-printed rib with tissue inserts in the form of silicone models. The rib cage is the same size as the term neonate's chest. Some have even taken the CT scan data of patients done for other reasons. This data is then processed in a 3D Slicer software resulting in a rib cage that will be an exact replica of the neonatal chest. (Fig. 12.2). The soft tissue for cutting and suturing is made from silicone. The strongest attribute for such simulators is the accuracy in terms of chest circumference and depth of tissue. The space limitation is also closely mimicked in these models. These high-fidelity simulators offer the advantage of doing the entire procedure of ligation of the fistula, division of the fistula, and esophageal anastomosis. Kathrine AB [5] presented a similar synthetic simulator; the neonatal rib cage models were designed in Computer-aided design software and then 3D printed as a composite structure. This essentially gives a high-fidelity box trainer which is not a box but an actual neonatal rib cage. Petra

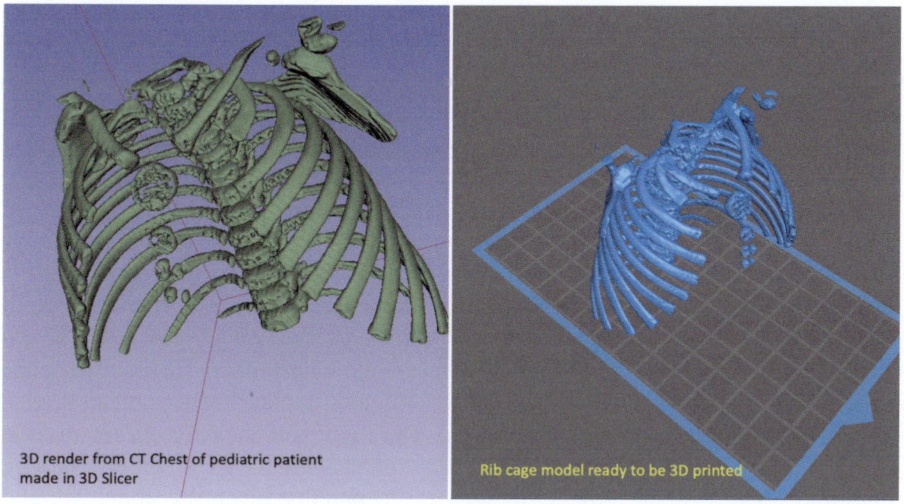

Fig. 12.2 CT render of neonatal chest made in 3D Slicer software. This can be physically printed as a scale model simulating neonatal thorax

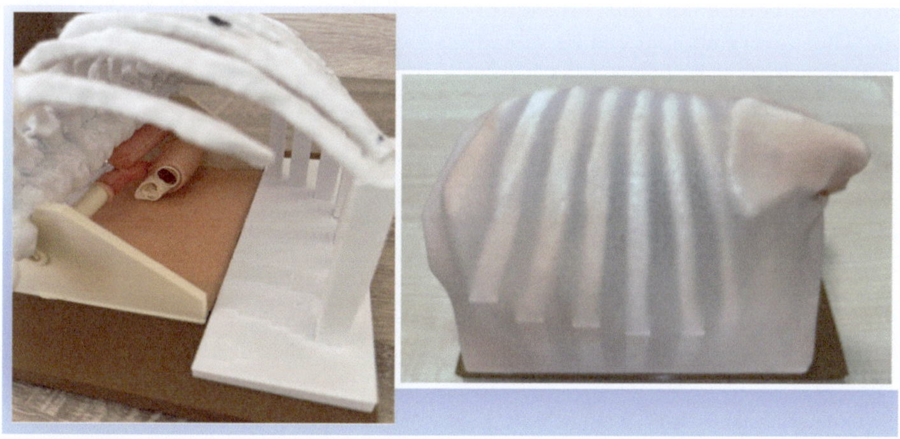

Fig. 12.3 Rib cage made from 3D printed material with synthetic tissue inserts made of silicone (image published under the Creative Commons Attribution License (CC BY) from open access article. Zahradniková P, Babala J, Pechanová R, Smrek M, Vitovič P, Laurovičová M, Bernát T and Nedomová B (2023)). Inanimate 3D printed model for thoracoscopic repair of esophageal atresia with tracheoesophageal fistula

Zahradniková et al. [6] used a similar mix of rib cage made from a mix of silicone and 3D-printed material to emulate the neonatal chest (Fig. 12.3). These models were validated though the users who rated the model with predefined parameters ranked on a scale like physical attributes, realism of materials, realism of experience, ability to perform task, etc. The advantage of such simulators is the low cost and the reusability of the materials once made.

In a review Nair D [7] listed the qualities of a neonatal minimally invasive stimulator on nine characteristics. These are low-cost, synthetic, disposable insert, scale model simulation, soft tissue textures, accurate replication of anatomy, accurate replication of procedural difficulty, collaborative design, and validation.

12.3.4 Virtual Simulators

In the era of advanced computing, virtual reality simulators or screen simulators provide high-fidelity simulation which can train surgeons through software. Virtual simulation is a computer emulation of a procedure on a screen without actual physical elements. It creates a three-dimensional image environment that can be interacted with in a real way. This is similar to computer games where you can drive a car with a real feel of driving and crashing. The flight simulator for airline pilots is a high-fidelity virtual simulator (VS) and can create actual case scenarios and rate the trainee. The VS can provide opportunity to practice technical, cognitive, and nontechnical skills under different circumstances. Newer versions of VS provide haptic feedback which markedly enhances the fidelity. These simulators also provide software-based objective assessment of performance based on parameters like procedural completion time, efficacy of motion, instrument clashing, force applied, etc. Thus, every attempt can be scored on a scale (Fig. 12.4). There are very few

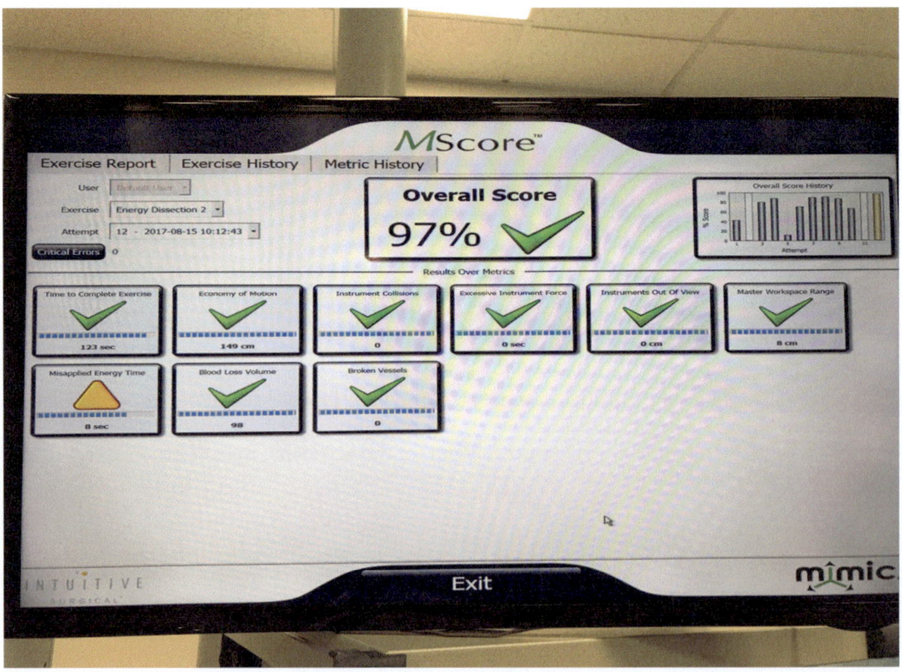

Fig. 12.4 Screen displaying score after a simulation exercise

Table 12.1 List of advance laparoscopy virtual simulators available in market for training in laparoscopy

S no	Parent company	Name of simulator	Country of origin	Remarks
1.	Laparo Medical Simulators	Apex Pro	Poland	Custom design to train for pediatric, **only simulator with TREAT as a virtual surgery**
2.	Surgical Science (Symbionix)	Endo Sim, Lap Mentor, Lap Sim	Sweden	Wide range of simulators for general surgery, endoscopy, and bronchoscopy
3.	VirtaMed	LaproS™	USA	Modules for general surgery, gynecological and colorectal surgery
4.	Medical X	LAP-X VR	Netherlands	Has mostly general surgery modules

pediatric-specific VS. Korzeniowski P et al. [8] developed a pediatric inguinal hernia repair simulator. Apart from other components, the input devices are the virtual Maryland forceps and graspers. These were validated using various parameters of user experiences. At present there are several advanced simulators.

Table 12.1 provides a summary of the currently available simulators. These simulators are not just available for surgical procedures but also provide simulation for other procedures like bronchoscopy, gastrointestinal endoscopy, interventional radiology, etc. The surgical procedure modules are widely available in these simulators, and new modules are being added as the wide adoption to these systems happens. These systems provide a very good preoperative warmup and rehearsal before the operation and increase surgeons' confidence in a low-volume center.

The disadvantage with these simulators is that they are extremely expensive to set up. The simulation of surgical procedure is close to reality and not real. The actual tissue feel is only in the form of instrument vibration as haptic feedback is still evolving. Not many pediatric-specific procedures are available. Most of the procedures are general and designed from adult perspective. Till the time of this writing, only Laparo Medical Simulators with Apex Pro had neonatal thoracoscopy procedure module available with these simulators.

12.4 Validation of Simulators

Deployment of simulators for skill acquiring and training cannot be done without validation. This is a process of establishing the truth value of a model and how accurately it represents the similarity to an actual scenario. Most of the time, this is established by survey of individual users at various expertise levels and rating the similarities to actual case scenarios on a percentage or a Likert scale.

MA Marcic et al. [9] used a similar system where groups of surgeons were made to perform various steps of EA-TEF repair. They were then made to rate the simulator model on a scale on specific parameters. These parameters were anatomical characteristics of model, usefulness of the model, and surgical anatomy compared to real anatomy. They concluded that >60% of surgeons rated the simulator model as high degree of similarity and more experienced surgeons completed the task faster than novices. This is what is expected in real case scenario thus establishing the validation of their model.

12.5 Rating a Trainee on Simulators

Trainee rating on simulators can be subjective or objective. Subjective ratings are done by mentor observation who evaluates a specific task performed. This method is cumbersome and expensive as it requires a set of people to evaluate. This is a classroom approach requiring full setup and schedule. Objective evaluation on the other hand is done by the computer software which will assess the trainees on specific predefined parameters. Some of the simulators developed have the ability of motion sensing and can plot the instrument movement; this is then compared to the ideal plot to rate the person. The software programs can rate on parameters as efficacy of movement, time taken, force applied workspace range, excessive instrument force, missed targets instrument out of view, etc. Oquendo et al. [2] detailed out specific simulator model with built-in motion-sensing capabilities. The advantage of such system is the versatility of practicing at any time or place without the need of mentor.

12.6 Conclusions

Simulation is essential for complex procedures. It reduces the incidence of complications and failures. Minimal-access training curriculum should follow the logical sequence of theoretical learning, simulation, and surgical apprenticeship and then finally allow to operate independently. Thoracoscopy and esophageal atresia repair offer extreme complexities, and students can be trained with the use of various simulators described in this chapter. There are several ways to rate the trainee with these simulators and grant him a license to operate independently or under supervision.

References

1. Barsness KA, Rooney DM, Davis LM. Collaboration in simulation: the development and initial validation of a novel thoracoscopic neonatal simulator. J Pediatr Surg. 2013;48(6):1232–8.
2. Oquendo YA, Riddle EW, Hiller D, Blinman TA, Kuchenbecker KJ. Automatically rating trainee skill at a pediatric laparoscopic suturing task. Surg Endosc. 2018;32(4):1840–57.
3. Narayanan SK, Cohen RC, Shun A. Technical tips and advancements in pediatric minimally invasive surgical training on porcine based simulations. Pediatr Surg Int. 2014;30(6):655–61.

4. Zimmermann P, Wiseman AX, Sanchez O. et al. The avian model: a novel and cost-effective animal tissue model for training in neonatal laparoscopic surgery. J Ped Endosc Surg 1, 99–105 (2019).
5. Barsness KA, Rooney DM, Davis LM, O'Brien E. Evaluation of three sources of validity evidence for a synthetic thoracoscopic esophageal atresia/tracheoesophageal fistula repair simulator. J Laparoendosc Adv Surg Tech A. 2015;25(7):599–604.
6. Zahradnikova P, Babala J, Pechanova R, Smrek M, Vitovic P, Laurovicova M, et al. Inanimate 3D printed model for thoracoscopic repair of esophageal atresia with tracheoesophageal fistula. Front Pediatr. 2023;11:1286946.
7. Nair D, Wells JM, Cook N, Moorhead A, Beasley SW. Critical design and validation considerations for the development of neonatal minimally invasive surgery simulators. J Pediatr Surg. 2019;54(11):2448–52.
8. Korzeniowski P, Chacon CS, Russell VR, Clarke SA, Bello F. Virtual reality simulator for pediatric laparoscopic inguinal hernia repair. J Laparoendosc Adv Surg Tech A. 2021;31(11):1322–30.
9. Maricic MA, Bailez MM, Rodriguez SP. Validation of an inanimate low cost model for training minimal invasive surgery (MIS) of esophageal atresia with tracheoesophageal fistula (AE/TEF) repair. J Pediatr Surg. 2016;51(9):1429–35.

Controversies and Contentious Issues in Thoracoscopic Approach for Repair of Esophageal Atresia

13

Contents

Learning Objectives

1. Application of thoracoscopy in patients with congenital heart disease
2. Thoracoscopy in low-birth-weight infants
3. Use of preoperative bronchoscopy
4. One lung ventilation for thoracoscopy
5. Use of clips for fistula ligation
6. Preservation of azygos vein
7. Primary posterior tracheopexy during esophageal atresia repair

R. P. Kanojia, *Thoracoscopic Repair of Esophageal Atresia*, https://doi.org/10.1007/978-981-97-5695-7_13

13.1 Introduction

Thoracoscopic repair of esophageal atresia is two-and-a-half-decade-old procedure. Surgeons have challenged this complex procedure's limits and gradually evolved, with more and more attempts being made in complicated scenarios. The growing evidence presented in the previous chapter has proven that thoracoscopic repair is comparable to conventional open repair and has similar success and complication rates. There is a complex interplay between the thoracoscopic intervention and the complex anatomy of esophageal atresia, which gets even more complicated by neonates' small size, emergency intervention, and anesthesia. Literature has deliberated over this complex interplay, and the best strategy for the neonate is yet to be established. This chapter discusses various factors associated with esophageal atresia, which can complicate and affect outcomes, and discusses the association and whether TREAT can be safely done in these conditions.

13.2 TREAT in the Presence of Cardiac Anomalies

Cardiac anomalies are a frequent occurrence with esophageal atresia. The incidence of associated cardiac anomalies is 30% [1]. These anomalies may range from simple conditions like PDA, ASD, and VSD to very complex cardiac conditions like tetralogy of Fallot's coarctation. Waterston's prognostic criteria [2] included presence of cardiac anomaly as a major factor for survival in these infants. In the past during evolution of TREAT, patients with CHD have been majorly excluded from the selection criteria for the procedure. This section will deliberate on the impact of congenital heart disease with EA and TREAT.

Pathophysiological Impact of Congenital Heart Anomaly During Thoracoscopy The anatomical surgical repair of esophageal atresia is no different in a patient with heart anomaly; however, the anesthesia and the effect of artificial pneumothorax produce significant physiological changes for the neonate while he is undergoing thoracoscopy. In open surgery the detrimental effect of pressure inside the thorax and the excess CO_2 is not present. In early experience most surgeons have excluded neonates with cardiac defects for this reason.

The positive pressure in chest has a twofold effect. First is because of the right lung collapse. The neonate is being ventilated on the left lung which is dependent because of the right lateral position. The lung compression causes more hypercapnia. This hypercapnia is increased by the absorption of CO_2. The hypercapnia in turn causes pulmonary vasoconstriction and pulmonary hypertension. This leads to strain on right heart and can cause reversal of the right-to-left shunt leading to desaturation. The hemodynamic consequence of the pneumothorax, on the other hand, will cause pressure on the superior vena cava and reduce the cardiac preload. This reduces the stroke output and can cause reduction in cerebral regional oxygenation level. The more severe the anomaly, the earlier and more detrimental are the effects of this phenomenon. This will lead to unstable patient with frequent desaturation. The anesthetist ends up hyperventilating with more pressure to wash out the CO_2. This may cause forced ventilation of the right lung which will hamper the surgeon's procedure by limiting his view. This at times goes into a vicious cycle and becomes a reason of inability to proceed with the procedure and ultimately conversion to open.

With growing science in anesthesia and better understanding of neonatal physiology, more and more series are being reported about thoracoscopic esophageal atresia repair with congenital heart disease.

Erika Fernandes et al. [3] reported nine patients who were operated with TREAT and had associated cardiac anomalies. The anomalies included five patients with VSD, one each of TOF, coarction, and ASD and three patients of valvular heart defect. They reported that presence of cardiac anomaly did not influence the outcome. There was no difference between the operative time between the cardiac and noncardiac TREAT. The gestational age was a significant factor associated with the longer operative time.

Christine Burgmeier et al. [4] reported a series of 15 neonates who were operated thoracoscopically for either CDH or EA. They had cardiac anomalies ranging from PFO to TOF. He concluded that thoracoscopy is safe in the presence of cardiac anomaly.

This brings us to the question of what cardiac conditions are there and which require cardiac correction before one can do esophageal atresia repair. Some severe congenital anomalies like tetralogy of Fallot with single-ventricle physiology, pulmonary stenosis, coarctation of aorta, and interrupted aortic arch are some of the conditions where a cardiac correction is warranted first and can be even combined with esophageal atresia repair.

In authors' experience, patients with cardiac anomaly are always considered for TREAT provided the anesthesia team is confident in maintaining the patient during thoracoscopy. The threshold for conversion is low if the patients desaturate more frequently than expected and if the procedure takes a very long time.

13.3 TREAT in Low-Birth-Weight Neonates

Thoracoscopic repair is a technically challenging procedure, and one of the factors making it difficult is the small size of the patient and the extremely small working space available. Initially surgeons at the learning curve of the procedure prefer to do a neonate who is good weight and is in good general condition. For premature and low-birth-weight neonates, the procedure presents additional challenges, and most of the beginners will exclude low-birth-weight neonates especially those below 2 kg. Carmen Dingemann et al. [5] proposed a criteria for selecting patients for TREAT they proposed a cutoff of 2000 gm as weight criteria. There are several studies for low-birth-weight infants and open thoracotomy repair for esophageal atresia. Data for the same set of patients is lacking for TREAT. Joonhyuk Son [6] reported a series of 41 cases of thoracoscopic repair where seven patients were below 2000 g. He reported that intraoperative factors were not different with the >2000 g group. There was no conversion to open in the low-weight patients despite having a higher incidence of congenital heart disease. There was no difference in the postoperative surgical outcome in the two groups. There is no other series available in literature specifically examining the association of low birth weight and thoracoscopic approach.

In general, low birth weight is not a contraindication for thoracoscopic repair. The prime factor for deciding the approach is the general condition and stability of the patient. Presence of associated anomaly especially cardiac defects is also affecting the surgeon's decision. Technically it is feasible, and success depends on the surgeon's experience and the anesthetic management.

13.4 Use of Preoperative Bronchoscopy

Use of preoperative bronchoscopy by the surgeon in esophageal atresia patients is done with the specific purpose of locating the fistula. The number and level of fistula can vary. From surgical perspective the surgeon must know if there is an additional fistula apart from the classic lower pouch tracheal fistula. Ten percent of esophageal atresia patients have an upper pouch fistula which is often missed. Preoperative bronchoscopy is however not done every time in cases of esophageal atresia as it is a time-consuming and equipment-dependent procedure. There are specific indications and targets for bronchoscopy in esophageal atresia; these are listed and described below.

13.4.1 Confirm the Presence of Fistula in Doubtful Cases

In certain rare cases, there can be gasless abdomen even in the presence of a fistula and the diagnosis can be confused with that of pure esophageal atresia. This can happen when either the X-ray is done too early in less than 4 h of birth [7, 8] or a narrow fistula gets blocked by mucous and epithelial debris and gas does not reach the esophagus to show normal gas pattern in the abdomen. In such cases a carefully done, rigid bronchoscopy provides valuable information about the presence of fistula and helps to decide the requirement of thoracic approach.

13.4.2 Confirm the Presence of Upper Pouch Fistula

Ten percent of cases with esophageal atresia will have an upper pouch fistula either as an isolated fistula or as an additional fistula to the lower pouch TE fistula. This is often missed in the latter cases as the attention is taken away by the lower fistula. A. Pigna et al. [9] reported 3 cases out of 15 who had pure esophageal atresia and had an upper pouch fistula. There are subtle clinical indicators which may point toward the presence of upper pouch fistula. The upper pouch in the absence of any fistula will have the distention stimulus intrauterine and will be a well-developed pouch; the gas shadow of the upper pouch will be sizable enough to give a clue that upper pouch is well developed, and hence there will be less chance of an upper pouch fistula. If the fistula is present, then this will lead to amniotic fluid draining into the lung, and the in utero distention stimulus will be less. This will also lead to excessive saliva pooling in the upper pouch to drain into the lungs, and this can present as a right upper lobe collapse on the chest X-ray. This specific location of right upper lobe pneumonia should prompt the surgeon to exclude an upper pouch fistula.

13.4.3 Trans-Fistula Guidewire Placement for Fistula Identification Intraoperatively

Some centers prefer to place a small guidewire through the fistula. This helps to identify the fistula during fistula ligation intraoperatively and assures that the surgeon is picking the right structure. The guidewire is removed once the fistula is looped. This is usually done in the early part of the experience by the majority of the surgeons. This is more useful for H-type variant of esophageal atresia; however, this is also reported for neonatal Type C esophageal atresia [10].

13.4.4 For Placement of Balloon Occlusion Device for Single-Lung Ventilation or Fistula Obliteration

Some centers have reported the use of bronchoscopy and placed a Fogarty balloon catheter to occlude the fistula. Peper VK et al. [11] did this with placement of trans-fistula Fogarty placement by rigid bronchoscopy. The Fogarty balloon was inflated and then pulled to occlude the fistula by blocking the esophageal side of the fistula. They reported the average time to place this to be 10 ± 2 min.

Similarly, Fogarty balloon placement can be done to aid in single-lung ventilation by blocking the right mainstem bronchus (Fig. 13.1). This will help to keep the right lung down during thoracoscopy and help intraoperatively. This if correctly placed and effective can act as a controlled on/off switch for the right lung ventilation. We have done this in the early part of our experience in the learning curve, and this helped reduce the ventilation struggles intraoperatively. This is however not preferred now as the Fogarty balloon stability is unpredictable and the positive pressure in the right hemithorax takes care of the right lung by pressure.

13.4.5 For Diagnosing Tracheobronchomalacia

One of the additional advantages of performing preoperative bronchoscopy is the early identification of tracheobronchomalacia (TBM). This can be a significant morbidity factor even after successful repair. Once we know the severity of tracheobronchomalacia, then intervention can be planned accordingly.

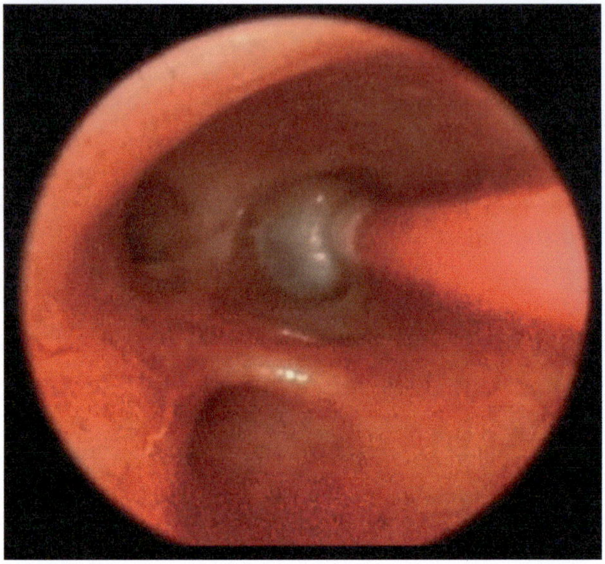

Fig. 13.1 Fogarty's balloon catheter placed in the right mainstem bronchus to occlude the lumen and control right lung ventilation

In a published IPEG survey [12] regarding the current practices during treatment of esophageal atresia, it was reported that 60% of surgeons did preoperative bronchoscopy. Nargis S. Ahmad et al. [13] published a multicenter audit of use of preoperative bronchoscopy in open and thoracoscopy repair. This was a nationwide audit from the UK. This study recorded 325 patients of which 25 were operated thoracoscopically. Out of the eight centers included in the study, the average percentage of cases undergoing preoperative bronchoscopy was 52%; of this 31% were done by the surgeon. This included flexible as well as rigid scopies.

In conclusion the requirement of bronchoscopy by the surgeon is to be judged based on the clinical scenario and the indications listed above. It should complement the surgical procedure appropriately. This should be actively discussed with the anesthetist and neonatology team.

13.5 One-Lung Ventilation

One-lung ventilation (OLV) or isolation of the right lung during thoracoscopy is not an absolute requirement. This is done with the aim to minimize right lung movement during thoracoscopy, so that accurate dissection can be done with minimum hindrance. In the early part of authors' experience when both the surgeon and anesthetists were in the learning phase, we started off with preoperative bronchoscopy and placed a Fogarty balloon catheter in the right mainstem bronchus

(Fig. 13.1). This was followed by regular intubation. In some of the early cases, where normal intubation was done, there was excessive movement of the right lung, and visibility was poor. Increasing the CO_2 pressure to get dissection space resulted in patient desaturation. This led to higher conversion to open. Occlusion of the right lung bronchus and thereby limiting its ventilation can help, and excessive CO_2 pressures are not required. We followed this in the initial ten cases and worked well, but this added to the operative time, and later with growing experience of both the surgeon and the anesthetist, we started doing more and more cases without single-lung ventilation and were successful. In a neonate with a good lung condition and no features of aspiration pneumonia on either side, single-lung ventilation can be avoided, and the neonate can easily tolerate CO_2 pressures of 4–6 mm of Hg. This is more favorable in the absence of any major cardiac defects.

13.5.1 Techniques of Achieving OLV

There are several ways of achieving single left lung ventilation. Use of Fogarty catheter has already been described in the above paragraph. The Fogarty balloon if properly placed in the right mainstem bronchus can effectively block the ventilation to the right lung and keep it quiet during thoracoscopy. The frequent problem of this technique is the dislodgement of the balloon from the required site during intubation and the requirement of rigid bronchoscopy for the placement. Another option is bronchial blocker, but these cannot be placed in babies below 6 months.

Selective left bronchial intubation is a challenging method to achieve OLV for right thoracoscopy but if achieved is most effective. In a blind approach, the endotracheal tube curvature is changed with the use of a stylet or a gum elastic bougie. The shape is given in a way that while advancing the tube during intubation, the tip will preferentially go toward the left bronchus. Figure 13.2 shows the angulation done for the tube before the intubation. This may take more than one attempt as it is a blind procedure. The confirmation can be done by disappearance of breath sounds on the right side with well-ventilated left side. Fiber-optic scopes which can travel through a 3 or 3.5 ET tubes are not easily available, but if available it can be used to confirm the position of the tip. Precautions must be taken to maintain the position while turning the patient lateral for surgery.

There are sporadic reports of this method. Ho AMH et al. [14] reported that left bronchial intubation in a neonate with right bullous emphysema was successful in the left mainstem bronchus. They used similar maneuvers to achieve this.

In conclusion, single-lung ventilation or right lung isolation is not required in all cases. This is more of the surgeon's preference and is also dependent on the experience of the anesthetist. The surgeon can keep this as an option in early cases to reduce the conversion rate.

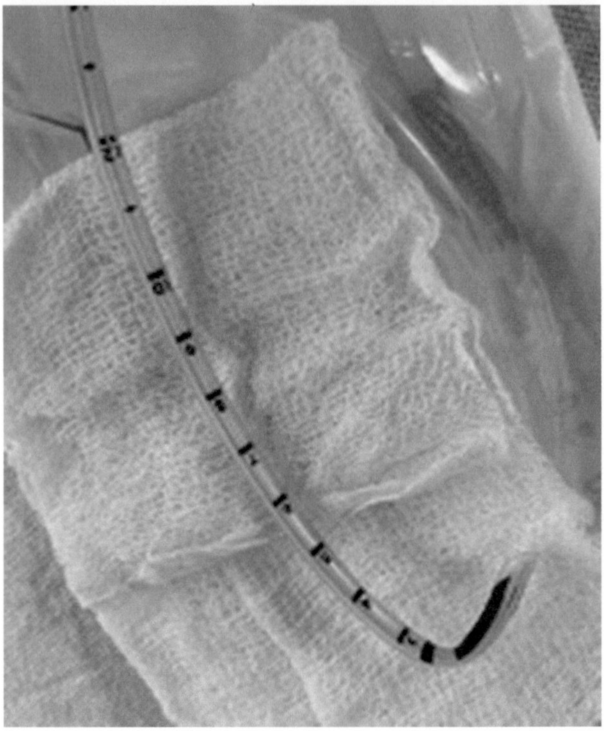

Fig. 13.2 Angulation done to the tip of endotracheal tube to achieve preferential entry into left bronchus during intubation

13.6 Use of Clips for Fistula

Ligation of tracheoesophageal fistula is a crucial step in TREAT. Ligation can be done either by nonabsorbable suture or by clips (Fig. 13.3). The use of clips in thoracoscopy is easy, saves time, and if properly placed achieves similar result as suture ligation. There are advocates for both suture and clips. There have been some reports of complications with clips being used. The most common is recurrent fistula and migration of clips. Schlesinger AE et al. [15] reported that after ligation of the fistula with clip, the clips vanished in the follow-up chest radiographs, and the patient had a recurrent TEF. The vanished clips were retrospectively analyzed as sign of clip dislodgement and trachea esophageal fistula. E Bindi et al. [16] reported as similar case of recurrent trachea esophageal fistula secondary to clips used to ligate the fistula. In their case the clips migrated to the esophageal lumen and traveled down to the stomach.

Chiarenza SF et al. [17] reported in a series of thoracoscopic repair where endoclips were placed in 28 patients, there were no postoperative complications except for intraoperative dislodgement in two cases which were managed uneventfully. They concluded that clip placement is safe and is a quick method although it requires a 5 mm port for access. No specific recommendation was made.

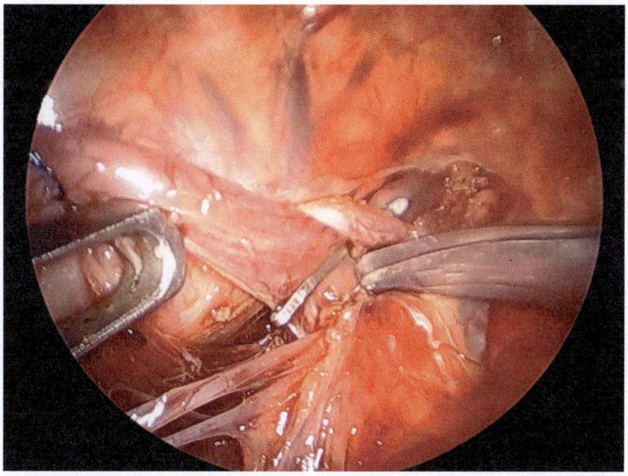

Fig. 13.3 Intraoperative picture showing fistula occluded by liga clip

In one of the largest series by Holcomb et al. [18], it was reported that out of 104 patients, 37 fistulas were suture-ligated, and the remaining had clips applied, and they did not attribute any of the postoperative complications to the clips application.

There is not enough data in literature to conclude if clips are safe, and it is up to the individual surgeon to decide on what he wants to use. In authors' own experience, although we did not have any major complication attributing to clips, we still prefer to ligate the fistula with suture trans-fixation as it is done in conventional open surgery. This is a time-tested method and is safe in the long term.

13.7 Preservation of Azygos Vein

The azygos vein is a major landmark, and it crosses and lies in front of the fistula. In conventional open repair, the vein is ligated for better visualization of the fistula and its separation from the trachea. In the last decade, there are many series in open repair which have advocated the preservation of the azygos vein and doing a more anatomical repair with anastomosis lying behind the vein (Fig. 13.4). The rationale behind the concept of preserving the azygos vein was that the vein receives drainage from the lower pouch of the esophagus along with some lymphatic channels. The ligation of the vein can result in more edema at the divided lower end of the pouch, and the anastomosis edge of the lower pouch will not be healthy and will lead to more chances of anastomotic leakage. During thoracoscopy it is extremely challenging to dissect the fistula and do the esophageal anastomosis with intact vein. With a skilled and experienced surgeon, this is achievable (Fig. 13.3).

Sharma et al. [19] reported a comparative assessment between two groups of EA-TEF with and without azygos vein ligation, and in their observation the leak rate was less in the vein-preserved group. In a systematic review and meta-analysis, Kainth D et al. [20] with six studies included in the analysis concluded that preservation of vein leads to less chances of anastomotic leak and stricture formation.

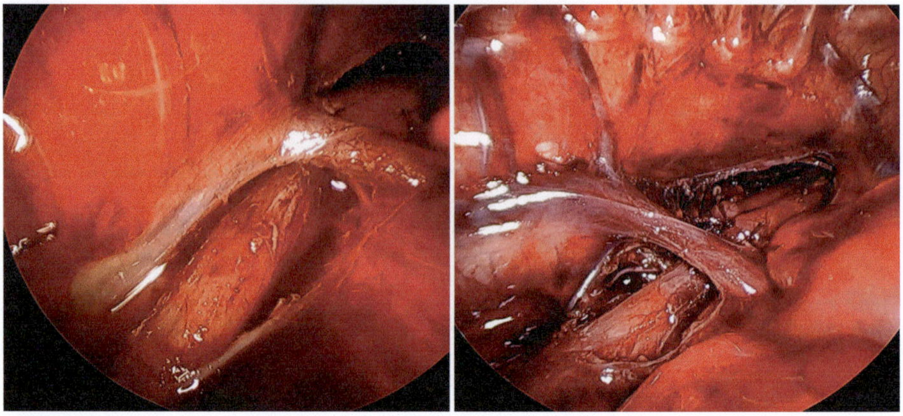

Fig. 13.4 Completed esophageal anastomosis with preserved azygous vein. Note the location of the azygous vein is below (medial) to the arching vein

Cui X et al. [21] reported 34 patients operated thoracoscopically and reported lower rates of anastomotic leakage and follow-up stricture formation.

The consensus is to preserve the vein as far as possible. If the surgeon can dissect the fistula and the pouches working his way around the vein without prolonging operative time, then preservation of the vein should be considered. However, if the dissection is difficult and the vein is hindering the view and dissection of the fistula, then the surgeon should not hesitate in ligating the vein. The ease of anastomosis is the priority, and if in any way this is made difficult by the vein, then it should be ligated. It is not an absolute certainty that ligation of the vein will cause more chances of leak.

13.8 Tracheopexy/Aortopexy during Thoracoscopic Esophageal Atresia Repair

Tracheobronchomalacia (TBM) is the segmental weakening of the tracheal tree due to softening of tracheal cartilage and hypotonia of myoelastic elements in the tracheal wall. This can be associated with or without esophageal atresia. Incidence of TBM with esophageal atresia is reported from 11–33% [22]. Treatment of TBM is well-known and is done by either aortopexy or tracheopexy. These procedures are established, and there is no controversy of doing them after the primary esophageal atresia repair is done. In recent time a thought has been raised that if there is a diagnosis of TBM with esophageal atresia, TBM can be dealt with during thoracoscopy. During esophageal dissection, the surgeon will have the opportunity of observing tracheal wall after he has completed the separation of upper pouch with the trachea. In the presence of a weak or floppy membranous trachea, the wall will be seen expanding and collapsing with ventilation. This is a confirmation of tracheomalacia. E Sofie van Tuyll van Serooskerken et al. [23] did a primary posterior tracheopexy suturing the wall of membranous trachea with the adjoining vertebral column in 14 patients. This avoided a second procedure, and in his series all these 14 patients had fewer episodes of respiratory infections as compared to another group where tracheopexy was not done. Akihiro Yasui et al. [24] reported the same procedure in eight patients with a lower incidence of respiratory complications.

In authors' opinion, if there is a floppy tracheal wall observed during TREAT, then a primary posterior tracheopexy should be performed within the same sitting. No additional dissection is required to do this, and at most two sutures are required between the tracheal wall and the fascia over the adjacent vertebrae. Care must be taken not to go through the tracheal wall as this may result in suture granuloma inside the tracheal lumen. This will avoid a second major procedure and a faster respiratory recovery.

13.9 Conclusions

Several controversial and contentious issues described in this text are subject to changes as per the evolution of the surgeon and his setup. Some of the comorbid conditions can be a contraindication when he is at the beginning of his learning curve, but later as the experience of his team becomes more, they will be able to handle cases like long-gap atresia, or atresias with congenital heart diseases. The same applies to low-birth-weight neonates. Other contentious issues like use of clips, preoperative bronchoscopy, etc. are a matter of personal preference, and nothing can be absolute about them. The surgeon has to develop his own preferences that suit him the best in his setup.

References

1. Chittmittrapap S, Spitz L, Kiely EM, Brereton RJ. Oesophageal atresia and associated anomalies. Arch Dis Child. 1989;64(3):364–8.
2. Waterston DJ, Carter RE, Aberdeen E. Oesophageal atresia: tracheo-oesophageal fistula. A study of survival in 218 infants. Lancet. 1962;1(7234):819–22.
3. Fernandes E, Kusel A, Evans S, Houghton J, Hamill JK. Is thoracoscopic esophageal atresia repair safe in the presence of cardiac anomalies? J Pediatr Surg. 2020;55(8):1511–5.
4. Burgmeier C, Schier F. Hemodynamic effects of thoracoscopic surgery in neonates with cardiac anomalies. J Laparoendosc Adv Surg Tech A. 2014;24(4):265–7.
5. Dingemann C, Ure BM. Minimally invasive repair of esophageal atresia: an update. Eur J Pediatr Surg. 2013;23(3):198–203.
6. Son J, Jang Y, Kim W, Lee S, Jeong JS, Lee SK, et al. Thoracoscopic repair of esophageal atresia with distal tracheoesophageal fistula: is it a safe procedure in infants weighing less than 2000 g? Surg Endosc. 2021;35(4):1597–601.
7. Gedicke MM, Gopal M, Spicer R. A gasless abdomen does not exclude distal tracheoesophageal fistula: the value of a repeat x-ray. J Pediatr Surg. 2007;42(3):576–7.
8. Goh DW, Brereton RJ, Spitz L. Esophageal atresia with obstructed tracheoesophageal fistula and gasless abdomen. J Pediatr Surg. 1991;26(2):160–2.
9. Pigna A, Gentili A, Landuzzi V, Lima M, Baroncini S. Bronchoscopy in newborns with esophageal atresia. Pediatr Med Chir. 2002;24(4):297–301.

10. Anderberg MBA, Stenström P. Transfistula guidewire for easier repair of esophageal atresia. MOJ Surg. 2017;2(4):43–4.
11. Pepper VK, Boomer LA, Thung AK, Grischkan JM, Diefenbach KA. Routine bronchoscopy and Fogarty catheter occlusion of tracheoesophageal fistulas. J Laparoendosc Adv Surg Tech A. 2017;27(1):97–100.
12. Lal D, Miyano G, Juang D, Sharp NE, St Peter SD. Current patterns of practice and technique in the repair of esophageal atresia and tracheoesophageal fistua: an IPEG survey. J Laparoendosc Adv Surg Tech A. 2013;23(7):635–8.
13. Ahmad NS, Dobby N, Walker E, Sogbodjor LA, Kelgeri N, Pickard A, et al. A multicenter audit of the use of bronchoscopy during open and thoracoscopic repair of esophageal atresia with tracheoesophageal fistula. Paediatr Anaesth. 2019;29(6):640–7.
14. Ho AMH, Flavin MP, Fleming ML, Mizubuti GB. Selective left mainstem bronchial intubation in the neonatal intensive care unit. Braz J Anesthesiol. 2018;68(3):318–21.
15. Schlesinger AE, Mazziotti MV, Cassady CI, Pimpalwar AP. Recurrent tracheoesophageal fistula after thoracoscopic repair: vanishing clips as a potential sign. Pediatr Surg Int. 2011;27(12):1357–9.
16. Bindi EGT, Noviello C, Simonini A, Torre M, D'Agostino R, Cobellis G. Recurrent tracheoesophageal fistula secondary to clips migration after thoracoscopic esophageal atresia repair. J Pediatr Surg Case Rep. 2020;62:101651.
17. Chiarenza SF, Bleve C, Zolpi E, Costa L, Mazzotta MR, Novek S, et al. The use of endoclips in thoracoscopic correction of esophageal atresia: advantages or complications? J Laparoendosc Adv Surg Tech A. 2019;29(7):976–80.
18. Holcomb GW 3rd, Rothenberg SS, Bax KM, Martinez-Ferro M, Albanese CT, Ostlie DJ, et al. Thoracoscopic repair of esophageal atresia and tracheoesophageal fistula: a multi-institutional analysis. Ann Surg. 2005;242(3):422–8. discussion 8-30
19. Sharma S, Sinha SK, Rawat JD, Wakhlu A, Kureel SN, Tandon R. Azygos vein preservation in primary repair of esophageal atresia with tracheoesophageal fistula. Pediatr Surg Int. 2007;23(12):1215–8.
20. Kainth D, Anand S, Singh A, Bajpai M. Impact of preservation of the azygos vein during surgical repair of esophageal atresia-tracheoesophageal fistula (EA-TEF): a systematic review and meta-analysis. Pediatr Surg Int. 2021;37(8):983–9.
21. Cui X, He Y, Chen L, Lin Y, Wang Y, Zhang J, et al. Clinical analysis of azygos vein preservation under thoracoscope in the operation of type III esophageal atresia. J Laparoendosc Adv Surg Tech A. 2020;30(4):448–52.
22. Corbally MT, Spitz L, Kiely E, Brereton RJ, Drake DP. Aortopexy for tracheomalacia in oesophageal anomalies. Eur J Pediatr Surg. 1993;3(5):264–6.
23. van Tuyll van Serooskerken ES, Tytgat S, Verweij JW, Bittermann AJN, Coenraad S, Arets HGM, et al. Primary posterior tracheopexy in esophageal atresia decreases respiratory tract infections. Front Pediatr. 2021;9:720618.
24. Yasui A, Hinoki A, Amano H, Shirota C, Tainaka T, Sumida W, et al. Thoracoscopic posterior tracheopexy during primary esophageal atresia repair ameliorate tracheomalacia in neonates: a single-center retrospective comparative cohort study. BMC Surg. 2022;22(1):285.

Cerebral Oxygenation During Thoracoscopic Repair of Esophageal Atresia

14

Contents

Learning Objectives

1. Understanding the impact of hypercarbia or hypoxia on cerebral oxygenation during thoracoscopic surgery for tracheoesophageal fistula repair
2. Role of noninvasive infrared spectroscopy (NIRS) in detecting cerebral oxygenation
3. Long-term neurodevelopmental outcome of intraoperative cerebral desaturation—evidence from literature

14.1 Introduction

Surgical repair of esophageal atresia is a neonatal emergency procedure. With the increasing use of minimally invasive techniques, thoracoscopy is now commonly done to approach this complex anomaly. During thoracoscopic surgery, carbon dioxide (CO_2) is insufflated into the thorax to collapse the right lung for visualization of the fistula and the atretic esophageal segment [1]. Due to CO_2 pneumothorax, there is an increase in the CO_2 load, over and above, produced by lung retraction

R. P. Kanojia, *Thoracoscopic Repair of Esophageal Atresia*,
https://doi.org/10.1007/978-981-97-5695-7_14

during open thoracotomy, leading to hypoxia, hypercarbia, and eventually acidosis [2]. In addition, there is a decrease in the venous return as well as hemodynamic perturbations because of elevated intrathoracic pressure and the anesthetic agents [3]. The above factors are well documented, and efforts are made by the anesthesiologist to prevent or decrease their occurrence by limiting the intrathoracic pressure used during thoracoscopy. Many studies have raised concerns regarding the impact of the above cardiorespiratory changes on the cerebral oxygenation and subsequent long-term neurological outcome [3–5].

There have been many studies on the effect of anesthetic agent exposure during the neonatal period on the developing brain; [6–10] however, studies investigating the impact of thoracoscopy on cerebral oxygenation have been few and with variable results [3–5, 11–15]. The measurement of cerebral oxygenation is not feasible with routine hemodynamic monitoring and therefore requires other sophisticated noninvasive modalities to monitor cerebral oxygenation. The commonly used cerebral blood oxygen saturation monitoring methods include measurement of jugular venous oxygen saturation ($SjvO_2$), brain tissue oxygen tension monitoring, transcranial Doppler ultrasonography (TCD), positron emission tomography (PET), and functional magnetic resonance imaging (fMRI) [16]. One of the new modalities which measure regional cerebral oxygen saturation ($rScO_2$) includes near-infrared spectroscopy (NIRS), which is used during the surgical procedure to optimize cerebral oxygenation and thereby protect the neonatal brain, and it has been the commonly utilized modality by many studies [4]. This chapter aims to present the available evidence on the effect of CO_2 insufflation on cerebral oxygenation, discuss the function and role of NIRS to monitor and assess brain oxygenation intraoperatively, as well understand how further research will help in improving the knowledge base for future favorable outcome.

14.2 Impact of Surgery and Anesthetic Agents on the Brain

Neonates undergo surgical procedures for a number of congenital anomalies. It has been shown in preclinical studies that anesthesia during the neonatal period is toxic to the brain leading to neuronal apoptosis or neurodegeneration in the developing brains of mammals, including rats, mice, and nonhuman primates [6]. This can lead to abnormal attention, learning and memory, and behavioral changes affecting the acquisition of higher cognitive skills [9]. It has also been shown in animal studies that the abnormalities are more if the duration of anesthesia is prolonged. However, how this translates into human clinical situations is uncertain and under investigation.

Since cohort studies would not provide any reliable conclusion, it was felt that randomized controlled trials would be useful in providing robust evidence whether general anesthesia (GA) will lead to worst outcome for the neurodevelopment. Based on this, an international, multicenter, randomized controlled equivalence trial was conducted in 719 infants of <60 weeks postmenstrual age undergoing inguinal hernia repair. They were randomly assigned to either a regional or general anesthetic group. The authors measured intelligence and intelligence quotient at 5 years of age as a primary outcome. The results of their study showed strong evidence that if infants are exposed to less than 1 h of anesthesia, then neurodevelopmental outcome is not different when compared to regional anaesthesia [8]. Although the GAS study demonstrated no difference in the intelligence quotient, however, it was not powered to assess the behavioral problems of the children. The impact of repeated exposure to anesthesia or anesthesia of longer duration was not assessed in this study and would require more research. Similar results were documented in the Pediatric Anesthesia Neurodevelopment Assessment (PANDA) and Mayo Anesthesia Safety in Kids (MASK) studies providing strong evidence that a short exposure to GA is not harmful to neonates [17, 18].

In studies assessing neurodevelopmental outcome after major noncardiac surgery during neonatal period, a mild to moderate effect on cognitive, motor, and behavioral function has been found [19]. There is a possibility that these changes are primarily due to GA or surgical stress causing hemodynamic, respiratory, and metabolic consequences [10]. Large prospective studies (GAS and Mayo trials) have provided no evidence of cognitive impairment in children of <3 years of age after a single short exposure to anesthesia provided they are healthy [8, 18]. However, major surgery performed in the neonatal period is generally of a long duration and may cause neurodevelopmental issues. This is because synaptogenesis, cortical pathfinding, and proliferation of oligodendrocytes take place during the neonatal period. Therefore, neonatal brain is more likely to be susceptible to harm than the mature brain of older children.

14.3 Impact of Hypercarbia and Acidosis on Cerebral Perfusion

14.3.1 Thoracoscopy and Brain Oxygenation

Thoracoscopic procedures in the neonatal period, because of absorption of CO_2 and a ventilation-perfusion mismatch, lead to intraoperative hypercarbia, metabolic or respiratory acidosis, and maybe cerebral hypoperfusion [20]. A decrease in cerebral vascular resistance causes an increase in blood flow and hyper-perfusion of the brain in presence of hypercarbia. In conditions of low oxygen saturation and a decrease in cerebral blood flow, cerebral vasodilatation caused by hypercarbia compensates the decrease in supply of oxygen to the brain [3]. It also causes a decrease in cellular metabolism and of high-energy phosphates, ultimately leading to acidosis. This activates enzymes and the transcription of apoptotic genes eventually causing cell death and neuronal injury. Insufflation of CO_2 into the pleural cavity, collapse of the lung, and reduced ventilation of the ipsilateral lung are responsible for all the above changes. In addition, the immature cardiopulmonary system in the neonate as well as the associated pathological disease can also impact cerebral circulation with harmful effects. However, till date the impact of thoracoscopy on brain perfusion or oxygenation and the long-term effects on brain development are unknown.

14.3.2 NIRS for Cerebral Oxygenation

The noninvasive measurement of cerebral oxygenation is required to evaluate the brain perfusion, and this is not a routine tool used in neonates undergoing thoracoscopic surgery. The most popular tool available for measuring cerebral oxygenation includes cerebral oximetry utilizing near-infrared spectroscopy (NIRS), measurement of regional cerebral oxygen saturation (rcSO2), and blood flow (rCBF) by a new device combining laser Doppler flowmetry and white-light spectrometry called "oxygen to see" (O2C) [16]. NIRS monitoring (Fig. 14.1) provides real-time information of the difference between tissue oxyhemoglobin and deoxyhemoglobin, reflecting tissue oxygen uptake and consumption. The rSO_2 provides information about oxygen demand, extraction, and reserve. Miyake et al. found NIRS to be a highly effective strategy for monitoring cerebral ($CrSO_2$) and renal ($R\text{-}rSO_2$) oxygen saturation in neonates and children undergoing minimally invasive surgery [4]. Below are the studies investigating cerebral oxygenation by NIRS in neonates and children undergoing thoracoscopic surgery. The authors recommended routine monitoring with NIRS to identify cerebral desaturation during neonatal surgery.

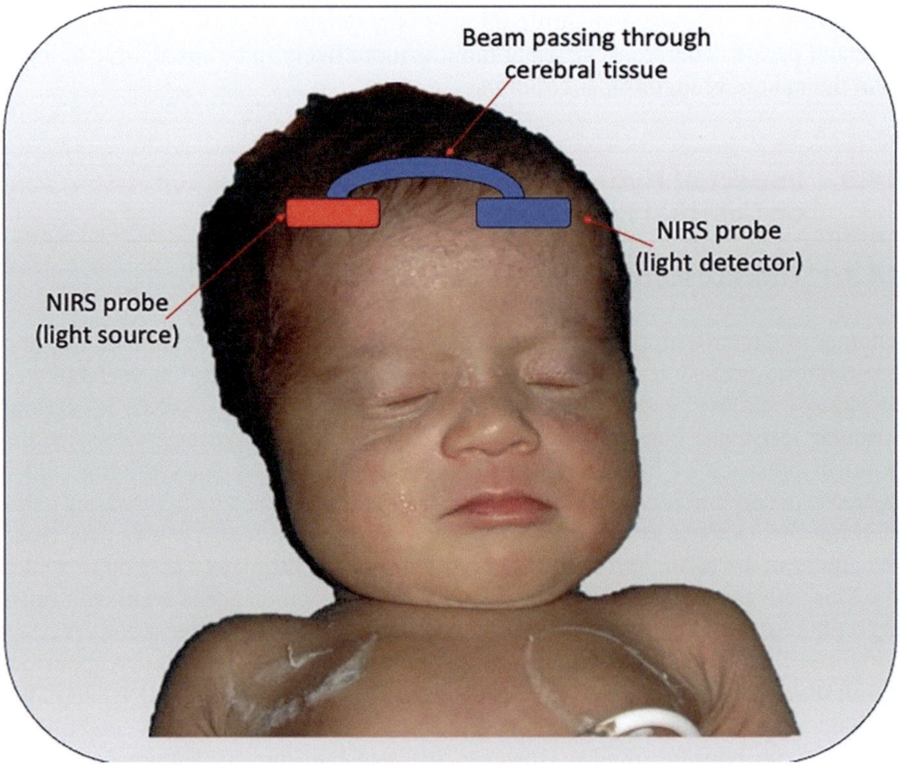

Fig. 14.1 Representative illustration on near-infrared spectroscopy for measuring cerebral brain oxygenation in neonates

14.4 Current Literature

Bishay et al. evaluated the effect of thoracoscopic surgery on arterial blood gases (ABG), CO_2 absorption (exhaled $13CO_2/12CO_2$ ratio measured by mass spectrometry), and cerebral oxygen saturation (regional cSO_2 by NIRS) in neonates suffering from congenital diaphragmatic hernia (CDH) and TEF [12]. They found that the thoracoscopic repair of CDH and EA-TEF leads to acidosis and decreased cSO_2. The absorption of insufflating CO_2 from the thoracic cavity was significantly more (29%). There was a decrease in cerebral SO_2 from 87 ± 4% (at the beginning) to 75 ± 5% (at the end), and this persisted till 12 (74 ± 4%) or 24 h (73 ± 3%) postoperatively. However, the authors suggested further studies to investigate the effect of hypercarbia on cerebral oxygenation and future long-term neurodevelopmental effects.

In another study by same author, the ABG values were compared in neonates undergoing thoracoscopic versus open surgery for CDH and EA. The authors found that the intraoperative partial pressure of carbon dioxide ($PaCO_2$) in the open group was 61 mmHg, whereas it was 83 mmHg in the thoracoscopy group ($P = 0.036$). The pH was 7.24 in open and 7.13 in the thoracoscopy group, and the time duration of hypercarbia and acidosis was longer in thoracoscopy compared to open thoracotomy group. The hypercarbia and acidosis were more severe in neonates with CDH. In patients undergoing thoracoscopic repair of EA/TEF, no significant difference in partial pressure of CO_2, pH, or partial pressure of oxygen (PaO_2) was observed [13].

With the aim of evaluating the effect of CO_2-insufflation pressure of 5 and 10 mmHg, on cerebral oxygenation and hemodynamic parameters, Stolwijk et al. conducted a research study in ten piglets [15]. The animals underwent anesthesia and were intubated and ventilated, and CO_2-insufflation was done using a pressure of 5 or 10 mmHg CO_2 for 1 h surgery. Animals were monitored for arterial saturation (SaO_2), heart rate (HR), mean arterial blood pressure (MABP), and $rScO_2$, and fractional cerebral tissue oxygen extraction (cFTOE) was calculated. Piglets receiving 10 mmHg pressure had significantly higher HR and MABP compared to the group receiving 5 mmHg. However, the two groups were comparable for $rScO_2$ and CFTOE. The increased duration of thoracoscopy affected the $rScO_2$ (increased) and CFTOE (decreased). The authors opined that insufflation of CO_2 with 10 mmHg pressure causes intense hemodynamic instability compared to 5 mmHg pressure. Higher oxygen extraction representing a decrease in cerebral perfusion may be a reason for this instability.

An observational study was conducted in 15 neonates undergoing thoracoscopic repair of TEF using 5 mmHg insufflation pressure. The authors monitored MABP, SaO_2, $PaCO_2$, pH, and $rScO_2$. Intrathoracic CO_2 insufflation caused a decrease in SaO_2 and pH and an increase in $PaCO_2$ which was reversible. At anesthesia induction the $rScO_2$ was higher, and it remained stable and within normal limits during and after the CO_2 insufflation, suggesting that thoracoscopy does not hamper cerebral oxygenation [3].

A prospective, observational pilot study was conducted to assess the cerebral and rSO_2 using NIRS, in neonates undergoing thoracoscopic surgery for CDH and TEF [11]. The neonates were monitored for HR, blood pressure, cerebral and renal rSO_2, ABG, and structured longitudinal neurodevelopment follow-up. There was no significant change in the mean CrSO2 during the pneumothorax (CDH = 82%, EA = 91% at baseline vs. CDH = 81%, EA = 79% at pneumothorax) in spite of severe acidosis (lowest pH 6.99). The neurodevelopmental outcome was normal at 24 months of assessment.

Abdallah et al. compared volume-controlled ventilation (VCV) and pressure-controlled ventilation (PCV) for their effect on cerebral oxygenation in neonates undergoing video-assisted thoracoscopic surgery (VATS) for TEF repair [14]. At baseline, the rScO2 was significantly higher in the PC group than the VC group, but it was significantly higher in the VC group after 15 min. Cerebral desaturation was significantly common in the PC group (80%) compared to VC group (33.3%; $P = 0.010$). To prevent cerebral desaturation, a higher fraction of inspired oxygen (FIO_2) and positive end-expiratory pressure (PEEP) was needed in the PC group. $PaCO_2$ was significantly higher in the PC group at 30 and 60 min. According to the authors, cerebral oxygenation is better maintained with VCV than PCV during VATS in neonates probably due to maintenance of a regular minute volume during the surgery. The similar cerebral oxygenation values during surgery may be related to the use of "volume-targeted" PCV mode of ventilation.

Neunhoeffer et al. evaluated the cerebral microcirculation, oxygen saturation, and oxygen consumption in neonates and infants undergoing thoracoscopy [5]. The authors utilized laser Doppler flowmetry and white-light spectrometry to measure $CrSO_2$ and blood flow. They also calculated the cFTOE and oxygen consumption. The authors observed a transient decrease (12.7%) in regional cerebral oxygen saturation, and this correlated with an intrathoracic pressure of >4 mm Hg in spite of a normal peripheral oxygen saturation. During thoracoscopy there was an increase in arterial PaCO2 (48.8 [36.5–65.4] mm Hg) and decrease in pH (7.3 [7.2–7.4]; $P = 0.008$) which recovered at the end of the procedure. There were significantly more frequent periods of $CrSO_2$ values <20% during thoracoscopy as compared to the control group. Based on these findings, the authors recommended that the intrathoracic pressure should not exceed 4 mmHg to avoid a decrease in $CrSO_2$.

In a 2023 systemic review, Prasad et al. assessed the impact of thoracoscopic surgery on cerebral desaturation in children using data from 7 studies (88 patients) selected out of 776 articles from 4 databases [21]. The cohort of patients included were mostly neonates undergoing EA-TEF surgery, and also included were children undergoing CDH and lung resection surgery. Out of the 88 patients analyzed, 13 (13.1%) of the children showed a significant desaturation. The mean (range) pCO_2 value in these patients was 72.6 (36.5–195) mmHg. Average pCO_2 values of 93 and 135 mmHg were reported by two studies representing significant hypercarbia [11, 12]. The $rcSO_2$ values ranged between 55% and 90%. However, the methodological quality of the included studies was limited. The authors have recommended that further randomized multicentric studies should be done to arrive at a definite conclusion.

14.5 Conclusion

Thoracoscopic repair of tracheoesophageal fistula is a rapidly evolving technique with comparable results with open thoracotomy. The effect of carbon dioxide insufflation on the respiratory and the cardiovascular system is well understood. It has been seen to cause significant metabolic and physiological alterations in the form of shunting of blood from right to left side, decrease in venous return and cardiac output, and hypotension and hypoventilation leading to severe acidosis and hypercarbia, which will eventually compromise the cerebral circulation. Various studies have used near-infrared spectroscopy for the measurement of cerebral oxygen saturation intraoperatively. However, the impacts of hypercarbia and hypoxia on the cerebral circulation and on neurodevelopment in later life are still debatable and under investigation. The studies done till now have failed to reach a definite conclusion since these studies have demonstrated that even with cerebral desaturation, the $rcSO_2$ remains normal. Therefore, one cannot make any recommendations for either monitoring or management options for this group of patients. Most of the studies done have small sample size and variable reporting, have included neonates undergoing multiple surgical indications (TEF, CDH, CPAM), and have failed to show any correlation with the long-term outcome of neurodevelopment.

References

1. Mukhtar AM, Obayah GM, Elmasry A, Dessouky NM. The therapeutic potential of intraoperative hypercapnia during video-assisted thoracoscopy in pediatric patients. Anesth Analg. 2008;106:84–8.
2. Szavay PO, Zundel S, Blumenstock G, Kirschner HJ, Luithle T, Girisch M, et al. Perioperative outcome of patients with esophageal atresia and tracheo-esophageal fistula undergoing open versus thoracoscopic surgery. J Laparoendosc Adv Surg Tech A. 2011;21:439–43.
3. Tytgat SHAJ, van Herwaarden MYA, Stolwijk LJ, Keunen K, Benders MJNL, de Graaff JC, et al. Neonatal brain oxygenation during thoracoscopic correction of esophageal atresia. Surg Endosc. 2016;30:2811–7.
4. Miyake Y, Seo S, Kataoka K, Ochi T, Miyano G, Koga H, et al. Significant neonatal intraoperative cerebral and renal oxygen desaturation identified with near-infrared spectroscopy. Pediatr Surg Int. 2022;38:737–42.
5. Neunhoeffer F, Warmann SW, Hofbeck M, Muller A, Fideler F, Seitz G, et al. Elevated intrathoracic CO2 pressure during thoracoscopic surgery decreases regional cerebral oxygen saturation in neonates and infants—a pilot study. Pediatr Anaesth. 2017;27:752–9.
6. Jevtovic-Todorovic V, Hartman RE, Izumi Y, Benshoff ND, Dikranian K, Zorunski CF, et al. Early exposure to common anesthetic agents causes widespread neurodegeneration in the developing rat brain and persistent learning deficits. J Neurosci. 2003;23:876–82.
7. Montana MC, Evers AS. Anesthetic neurotoxicity: new findings and future directions. J Pediatr. 2017;181:279–85.
8. McCann ME, de Graaff JC, Dorris L, Disma N, Withington D, Bell G, et al. Neurodevelopmental outcome at 5 years of age after general anaesthesia or awake- regional anaesthesia in infancy (GAS): an international, multicentre, randomised controlled equivalence trial. Lancet. 2019;393:664–77.
9. Keunen K, Weiland NHS, de Bakker BS, de Vries LS, Stevens MF. Impact of surgery and anesthesia during early brain development: a perfect storm. Paediatr Anaesth. 2022;32:697–705.

10. Stolwijk LJ, Lemmers MA, Harmsen M. Neurodevelopmental outcomes after neonatal surgery for major noncardiac anomalies. Pediatrics. 2016;137:e20151728.
11. Costerus S, Vlot J, van Rosmalen J, Wijnen R, Weber F. Effects of neonatal thoracoscopic surgery on tissue oxygenation: a pilot study on (neuro-) monitoring and outcomes. Eur J Pediatr Surg. 2019;29:166–72.
12. Bishay M, Giacomello L, Retrosi G, Nah MTSA, McHoney M, Coppi PD, et al. Decreased cerebral oxygen saturation during thoracoscopic repair of congenital diaphragmatic hernia and esophageal atresia in infants. J Pediatr Surg. 2011;46:47–51.
13. Bishay M, Giacomello L, Retrosi G, Thyoka M, Garriboli M, Brierley J, et al. Hypercapnia and acidosis during open and thoracoscopic repair of congenital diaphragmatic hernia and esophageal atresia. Results of a pilot randomized controlled trial. Ann Surg. 2013;258:895–900.
14. Abdallah NM, Elela A, Maghawry HH, Alkonaiesy RM. Effect of different mechanical ventilation modes on cerebral blood flow during thoracoscopic surgery in neonates: a randomised controlled trial. Indian J Anaesth. 2022;66:651–6.
15. Stolwijk LJ, Tytgat SHAJ, Keunen K, Suksamanapan N, van Herwaarden MYA, Groenendaal F, et al. The effects of CO2-insufflation with 5 and 10 mmHg during thoracoscopy on cerebral oxygenation and hemodynamics in piglets: an animal experimental study. Surg Endosc. 2015;29:2781–8.
16. Kirkman MA, Smith M. Brain oxygenation monitoring. Anesthesiol Clin. 2016;34:537–56.
17. Sun LS, Li G, Miller TL, Salorio C, Byrne MW, Bellinger DC, et al. Association between a single general anesthesia exposure before age 36 months and neurocognitive outcomes in later childhood. JAMA. 2016;315:2312–20.
18. Warner DO, Zaccariello MJ, Katusic SK, Schroeder DR, Hanson AC, Schulte PJ, et al. Neuropsychological and behavioral outcomes after exposure of young children to procedures requiring general anesthesia: the Mayo Anesthesia Safety in Kids (MASK) study. Anesthesiology. 2018;129:89–105.
19. Stolwijk LJ, Keunen K, De Vries LS, Groenendaal F, van der Zee DC, van Herwaarden MYA, et al. Neonatal surgery for noncardiac congenital anomalies: neonates at risk of brain injury. J Pediatr. 2016;182:335–41.e1
20. Pierro A. Hypercapnia and acidosis during the thoracoscopic repair of oesophageal atresia and congenital diaphragmatic hernia. J Pediatr Surg. 2015;50:247–9.
21. Prasad G, Singh A, Kainth D, Khanna P, Anand S. Intraoperative regional cerebral oxygenation during pediatric thoracoscopic surgery: a systematic review. J Laparoendosc Adv Surg Tech A. 2023; https://doi.org/10.1089/lap.2023.0228. Online ahead of print

Thoracoscopic Repair of Esophageal Atresia: Pictorial Essay

15

Contents

15.1 Introduction

Thoracoscopic repair of esophageal atresia is a technically demanding procedure with long learning curve. This book presents an extensive description of esophageal management with thoracoscopy to help with the learning curve. Starting from anatomy, case selection patient positioning, port placement, and detailed steps of

R. P. Kanojia, *Thoracoscopic Repair of Esophageal Atresia*, https://doi.org/10.1007/978-981-97-5695-7_15

surgery are presented. Classic EA-TEF as well as variations are described for better understanding. For a beginner, it is essential to have a road map in the mind when he is making his first few attempts. A mental run through via pictures and videos helps in anticipating problems and preparing the team for the procedure. Nothing says more than a picture for quickly recapitulating the steps of surgery. This chapter presents a pictographic depiction of TREAT from start to finish. Going through the sequential pictures of TREAT before the surgery will help the surgeon to pick up pace and keep his motivation alive as he progresses intra-operatively and keeps matching the mental image with what he sees on screen.

15.2 Radiology

Chest X-ray is one of the deciding factors for patient selection. Findings on the plain X-ray should be carefully evaluated to see if thoracoscopy is safely feasible (Figs. 15.1, 15.2 and 15.3).

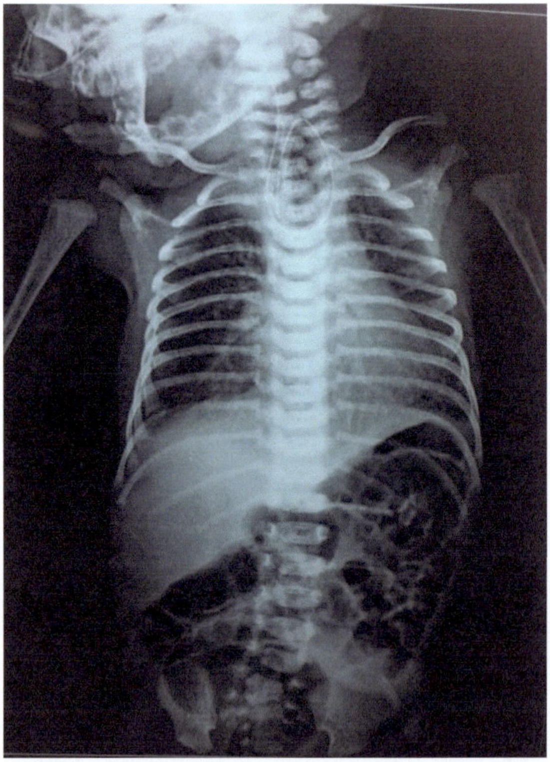

Fig. 15.1 Plain Chest X-ray showing feeding tube coiling at the level of T3-T4. The assessment to be made on X-ray is the level of pouch. Note the sacral hemivertebrae and 13 pair of ribs. Extra rib is an indication to look for other VACTERL anomalies and expect a long gap atresia. Note the good gas pattern in abdomen with small gastric bubble indicating a narrow fistula

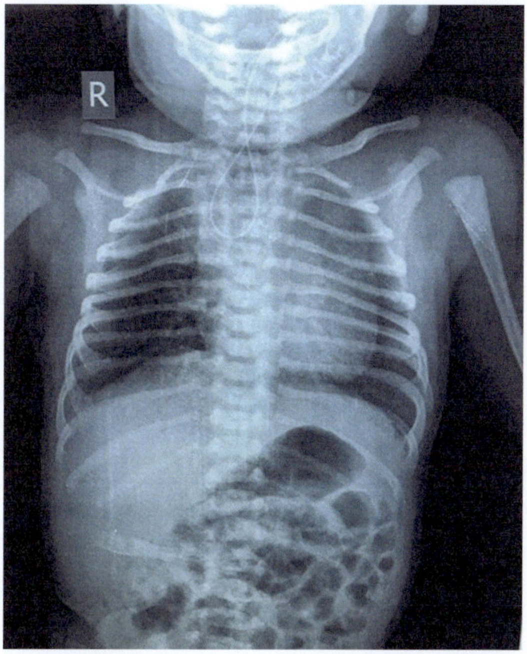

Fig. 15.2 Another example of chest X-ray showing coiling of tube and abnormally enlarged heart shadow. This patient will need to be evaluated for cardiac anomalies and can be a high-risk patient for thoracoscopy

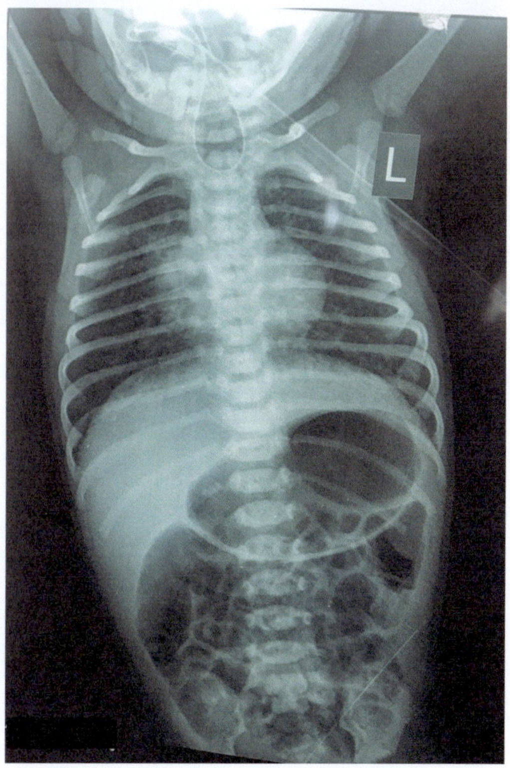

Fig. 15.3 Chest X-ray showing a high coiling of feeding tube in upper pouch. This may be a long gap esophageal atresia, and difficulty during primary anastomosis can be anticipated with higher chance of conversion to open or esophageal diversion

15.3 Operation Theater Layout

See Fig. 15.4.

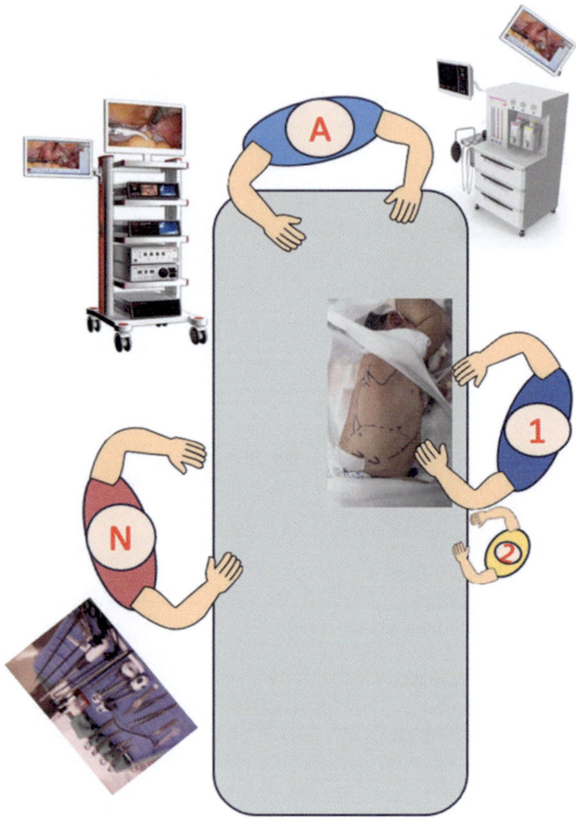

Fig. 15.4 Operation theater layout: General layout of operation theater during TREAT. Note how the neonate is positioned on the left edge of the table closer to the surgeon with the surgeon maintaining a straight line between surgeon-camera-organ-picture (SCOP). The anesthetist has his own surgical monitor within his comfort zone so that he watches and synchronizes with surgical steps

15.4 Patient Positioning

See Figs. 15.5 and 15.6.

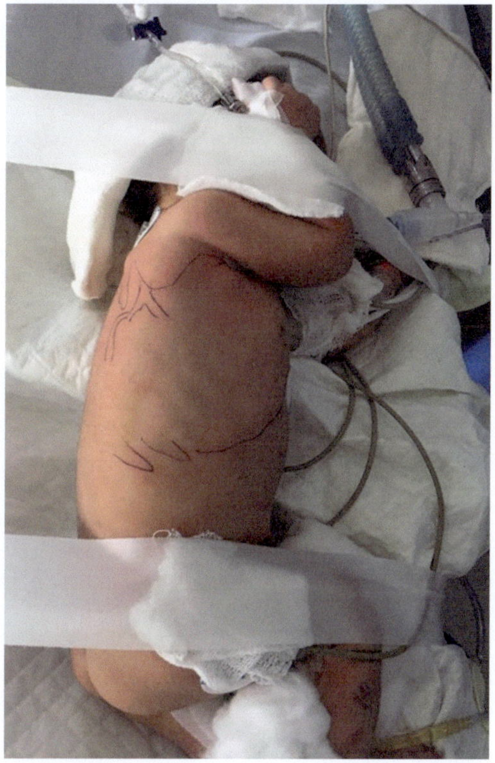

Fig. 15.5 Neonate positioned on table and strapped for stability. Detailed description on how to position is described in Chap. 5. Note that this is a three-quarter semi-prone position and the degree of making him prone can be modified with additional table tilt

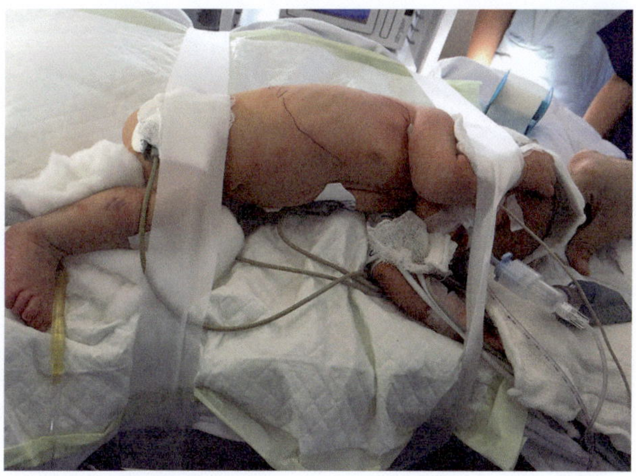

Fig. 15.6 Neonate's position viewed from side. Note the soft roll under the rib cage to elevate the right hemithorax

15.5 Surface Markings and Port Positions

See Figs. 15.7 and 15.8.

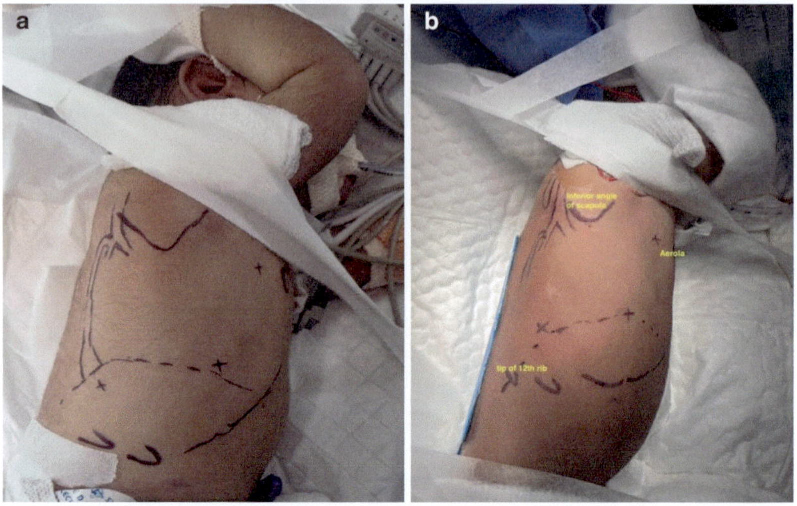

Fig. 15.7 (**a**, **b**) l: Landmarks for port placement. Areola, tip of 12th rib, and inferior angle of scapula are three most important landmarks. Note the surface anatomy drawn for diaphragm, lowermost ribs, and the presumed position of upper pouch and fistula

Fig. 15.8 Surface markings and markings for port showing how good triangularization can be achieved with knowledge of surface anatomy

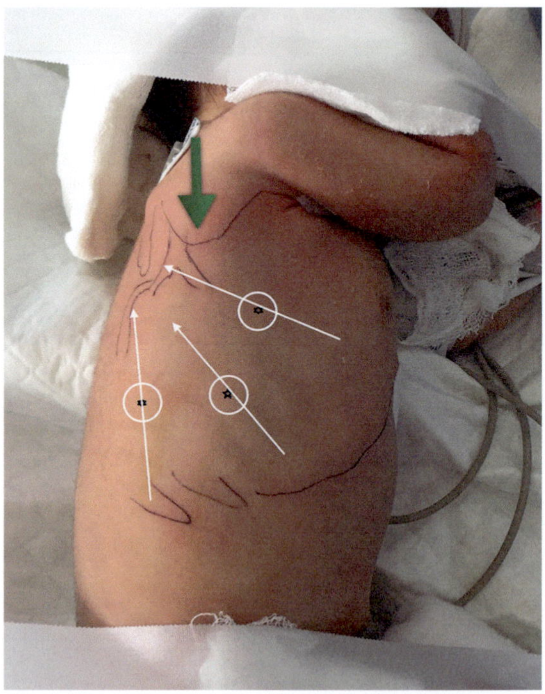

15.6 Steps of Thoracoscopic Repair of Esophageal Atresia with Type C Anatomy

See Figs. 15.9 and 15.10.

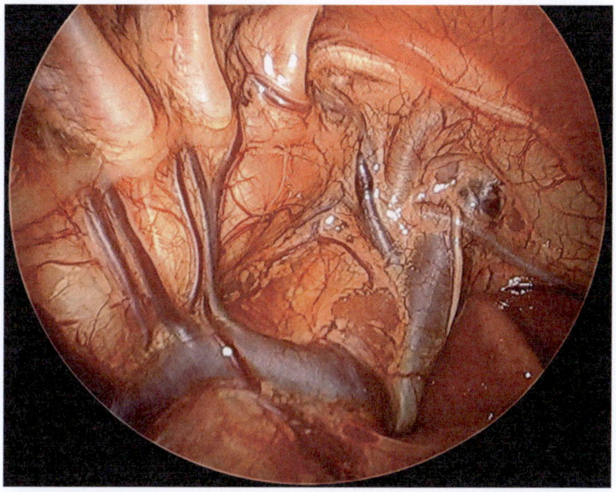

Fig. 15.9 Initial anatomy of right hemithorax seen during thoracoscopy

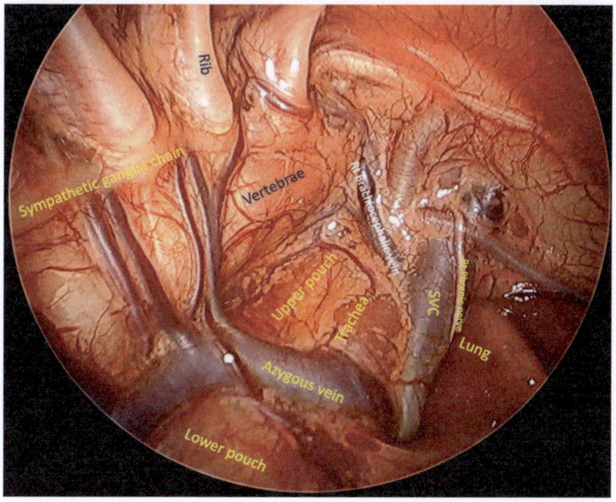

Fig. 15.10 Labeled anatomy for above image

15.7 Lower Pouch Identification

See Fig. 15.11.

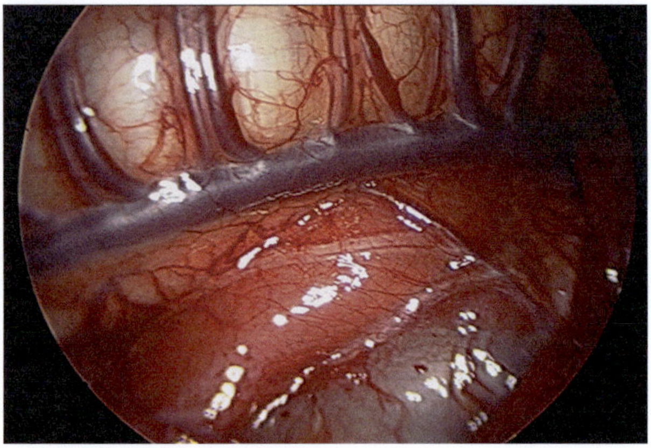

Fig. 15.11 Lower pouch is identified by the synchronized distention of the fistula. Also note the vagus running over the lower pouch of esophagus

15.8 Azygous Vein Division

See Fig. 15.12.

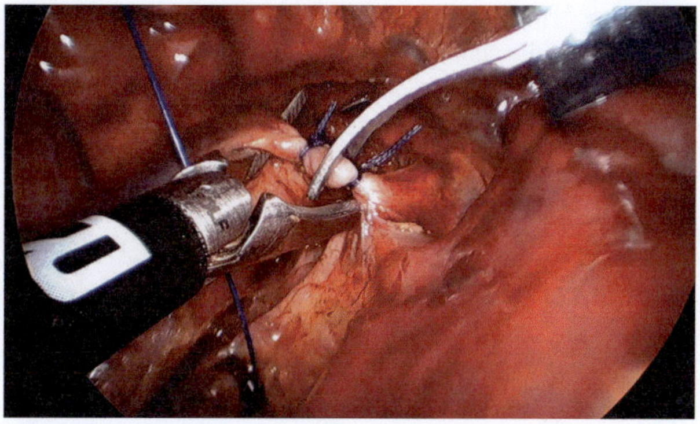

Fig. 15.12 Azygous vein can be ligated with 2 free ties and then divided in between. Alternatively harmonic scalpel or any other vessel sealing device can be used

15.9 Chest Wall Hitch for Dissecting Fistula

See Figs. 15.13 and 15.14.

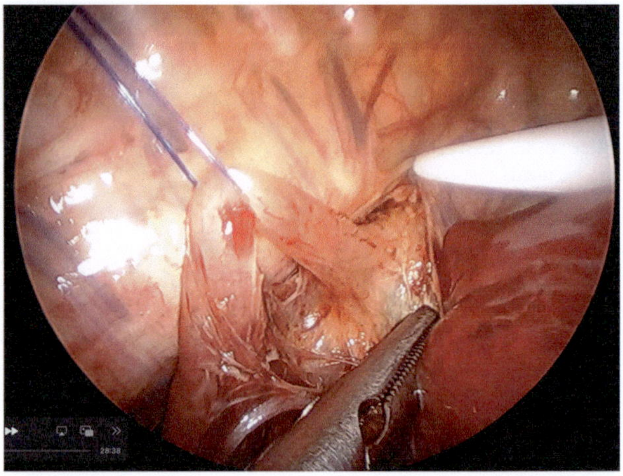

Fig. 15.13 The lower pouch is looped around a prolene hitch stitch. This helps to lift up the fistula and precisely see the tracheo-esophageal fistula junction

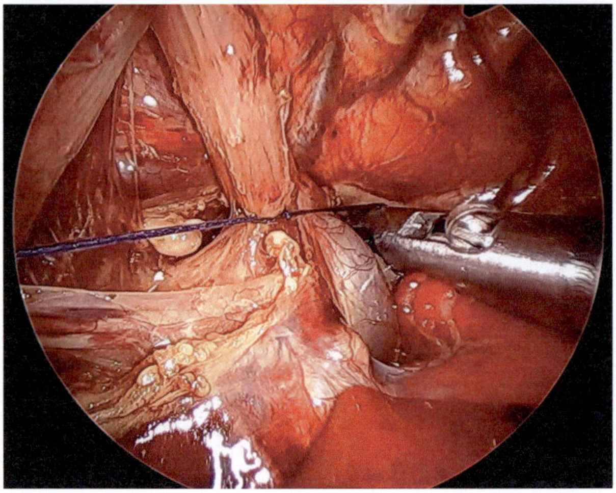

Fig. 15.14 Trans fixation and ligation of fistula. Note the hitch stich is helping to lift up the lower pouch

15.10 Mobilization of Upper Pouch

See Figs. 15.15 and 15.16.

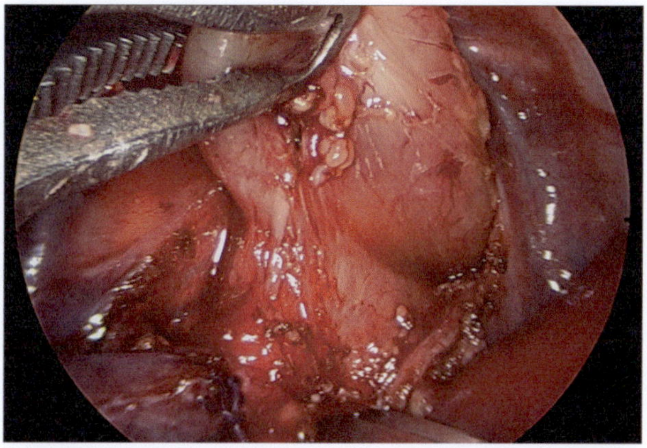

Fig. 15.15 Upper pouch is in close association with trachea and needs to be dissected off it so that gain in length is there for easy anastomosis. The figure shows the plane between the two

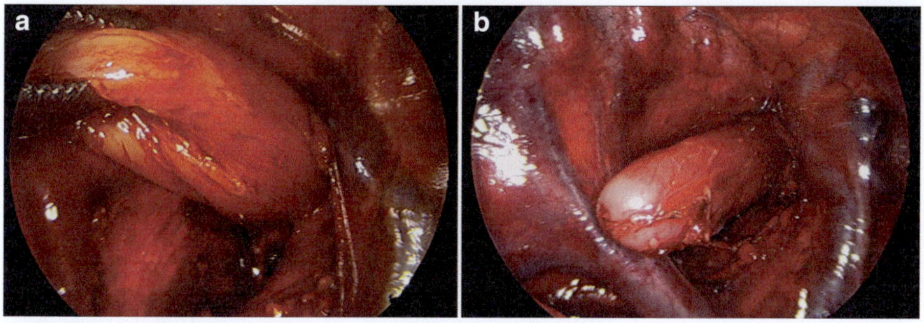

Fig. 15.16 Upper pouch is now seen completely separated from tracheal side (**a**), and with the push of upper pouch feeding tube, it can move down to level of azygous vein (**b**) indicating tension-free anastomosis

15.11 Opening of Upper Pouch before Starting Anastomosis

See Figs. 15.17 and 15.18.

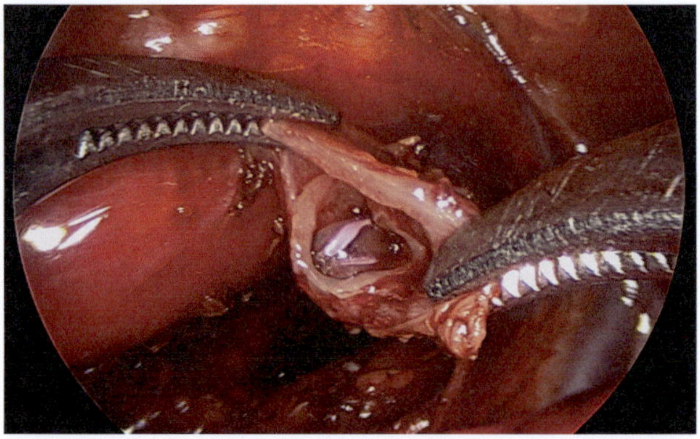

Fig. 15.17 Upper pouch is opened over the tip of feeding tube to open the lumen. Note how the mucosa recedes after cutting

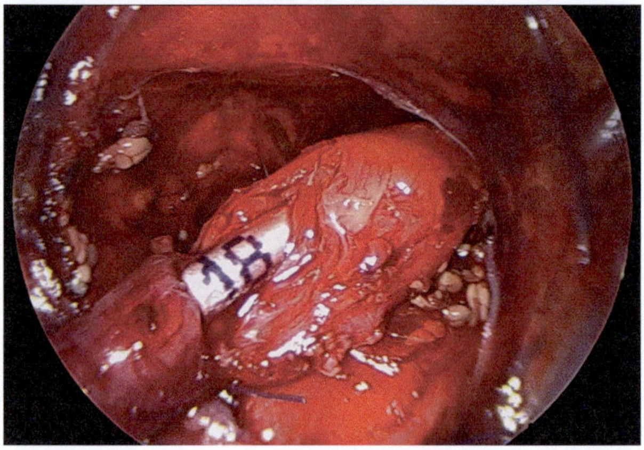

Fig. 15.18 Posterior layer of anastomosis completed with the trans-anastomotic tube in place

15.12 Completed Anastomosis

See Figs. 15.19 and 15.20.

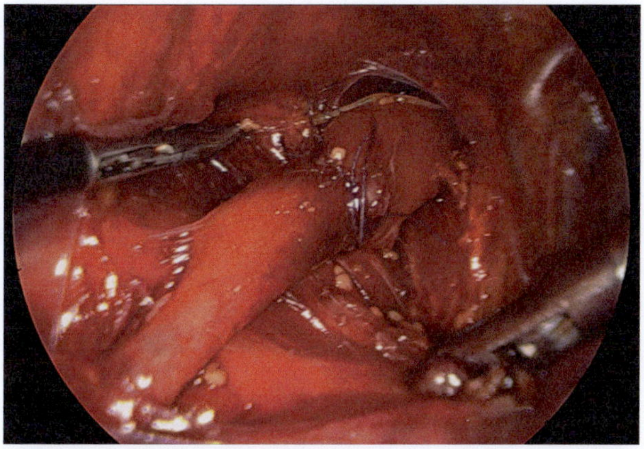

Fig. 15.19 Completed anastomosis with final view. Note that the azygous vein has been ligated in this case

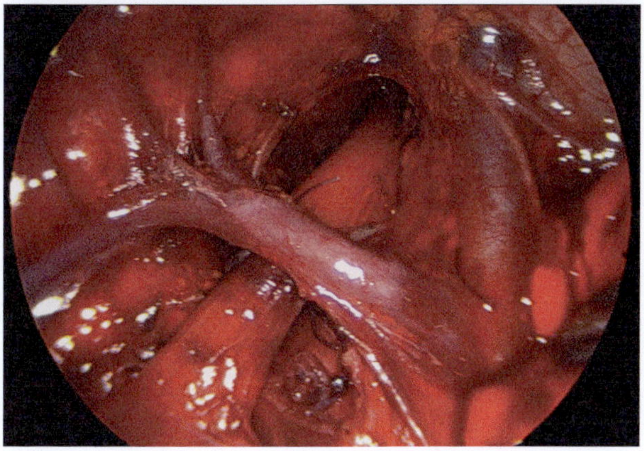

Fig. 15.20 Completed anastomosis with preservation of azygous vein. Note that the anastomosis lies behind the vein in natural position

15.13 Postoperative Esophagogram

See Figs. 15.21, 15.22 and 15.23.

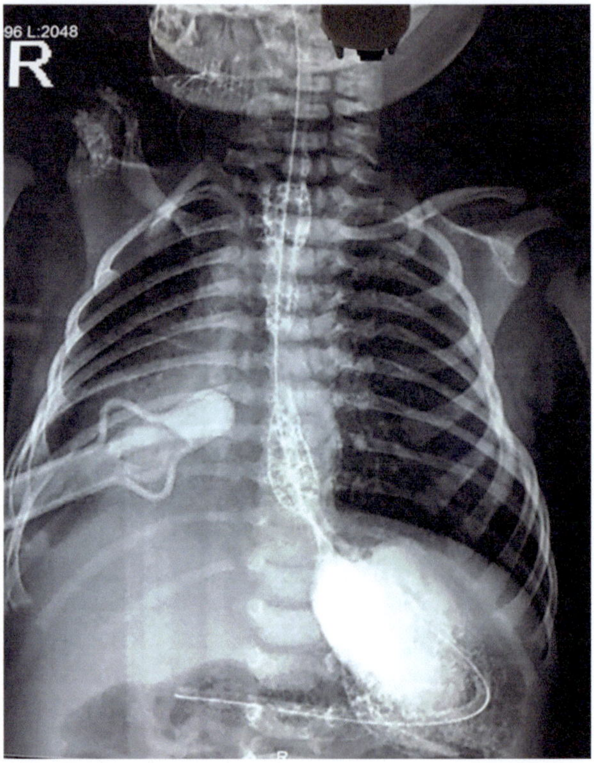

Fig. 15.21 Contrast esophagogram showing normal passage of dye with normal anastomotic caliber

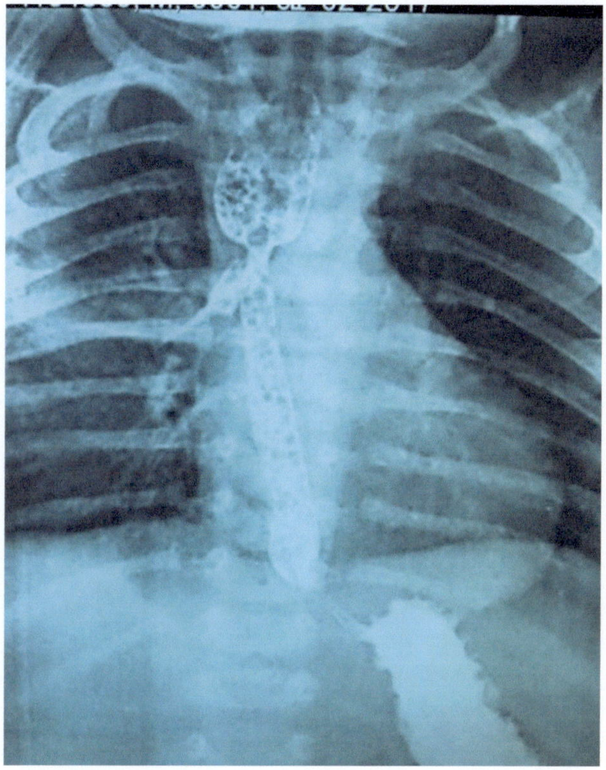

Fig. 15.22 Contrast esophagogram showing minor leak at the anastomotic site. This can be managed conservatively

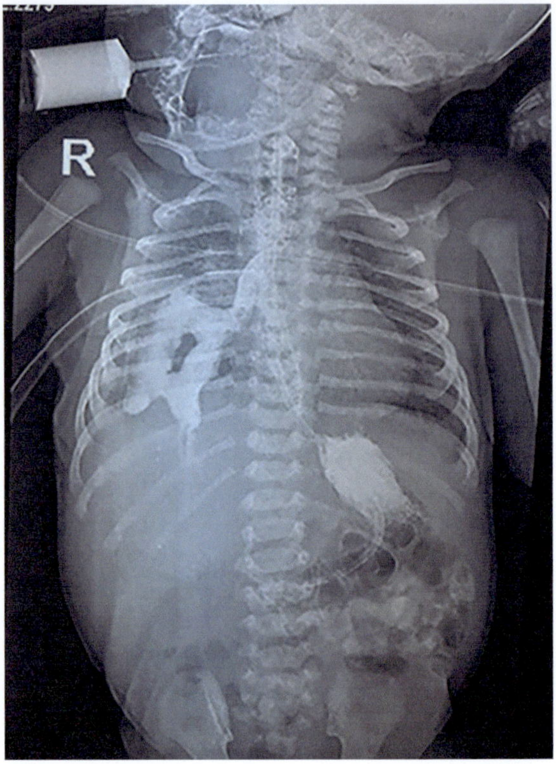

Fig. 15.23 Major leak with dye freely going into mediastinum

15.14 Esophageal Stricture After TREAT

See Figs. 15.24 and 15.25.

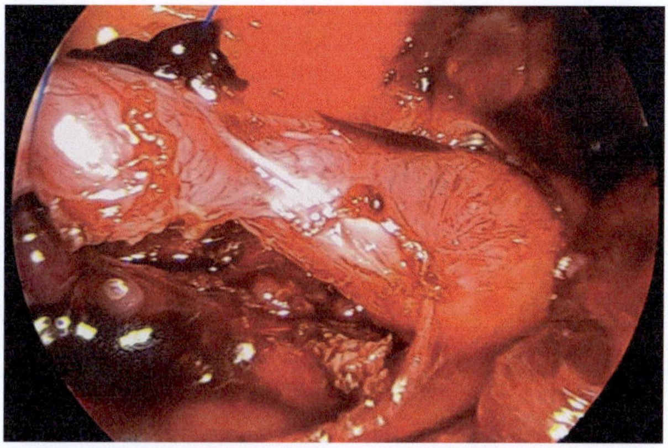

Fig. 15.24 Thoracoscopic view of esophageal stricture after previous TREAT. Several attempts at dilatation failed in this patient

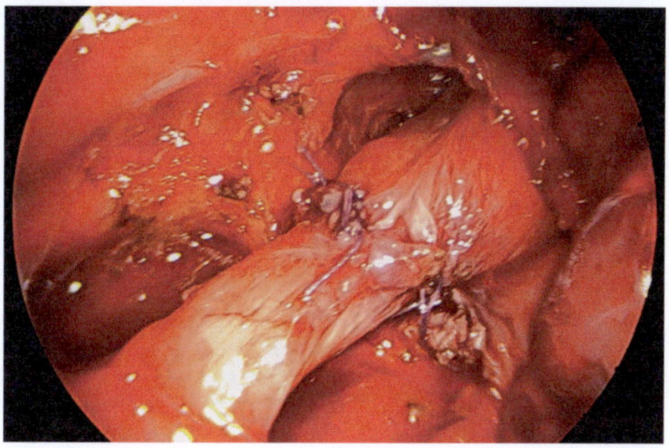

Fig. 15.25 Same as above figure after complete excision of stricture and redo anastomosis

15.15 Thoracoscopic Repair in Esophageal Atresia with Right Aortic Arch

See Figs. 15.26 and 15.27.

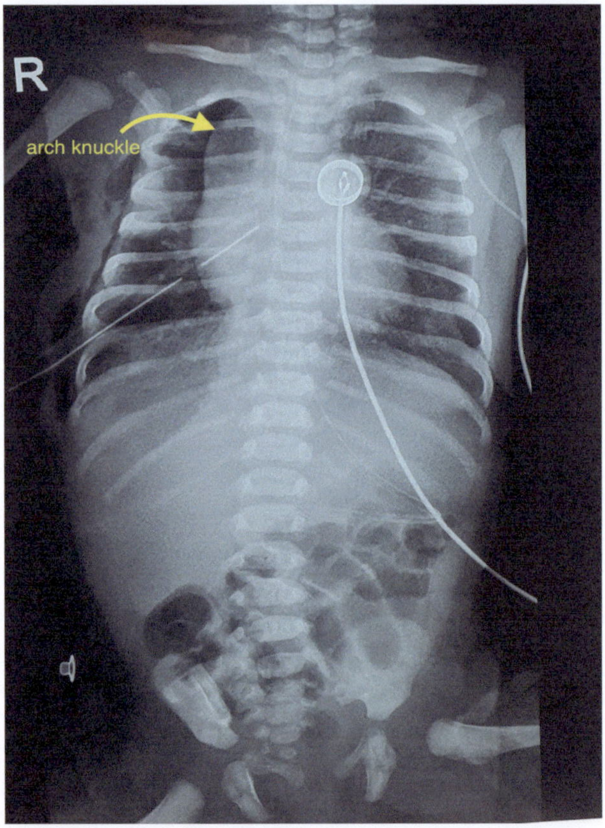

Fig. 15.26 Preoperative X-ray in a patient with right aortic arch showing the curve of the aortic arch

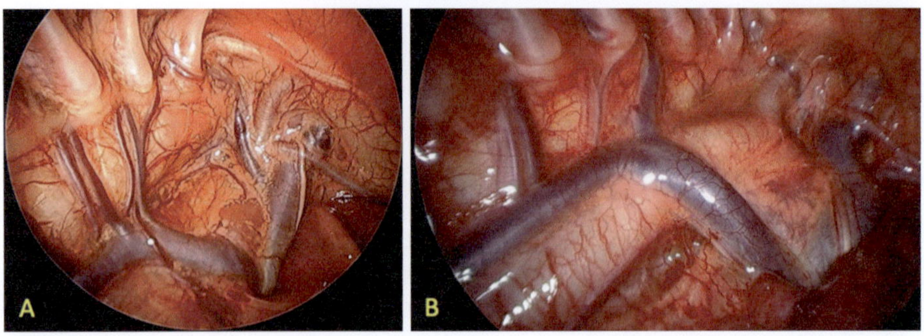

Fig. 15.27 Comparative anatomy between a classic esophageal atresia (**a**) and one with RAA. Note how the aorta is prominently seen (**b**)

15.16 Other Vascular Aberrations

See Figs. 15.28 and 15.29.

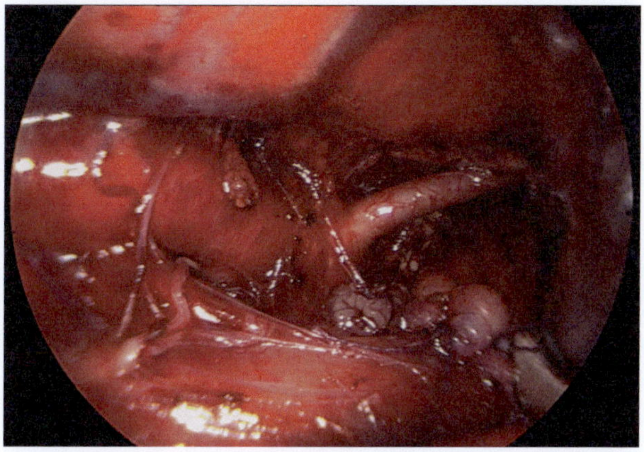

Fig. 15.28 Aberrant right subclavian vessel can be seen originating from the arch and going to the left side

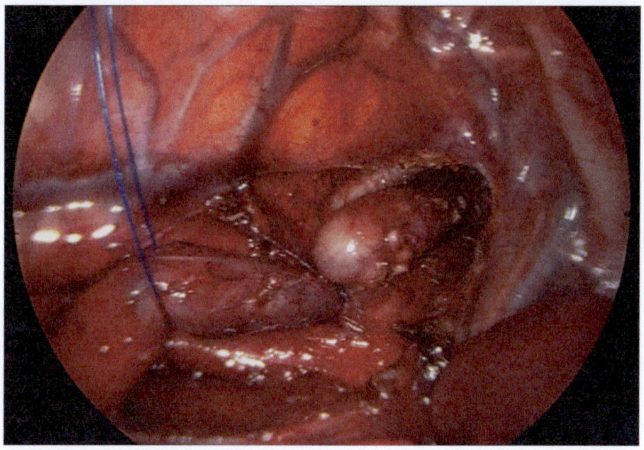

Fig. 15.29 Aberrant right subclavian vessel can be seen next to the upper pouch and can be injured during the upper pouch mobilization if the surgeon is unaware of it

15.17 Recurrent Tracheo-Esophageal Fistula After TREAT

See Figs. 15.30 and 15.31.

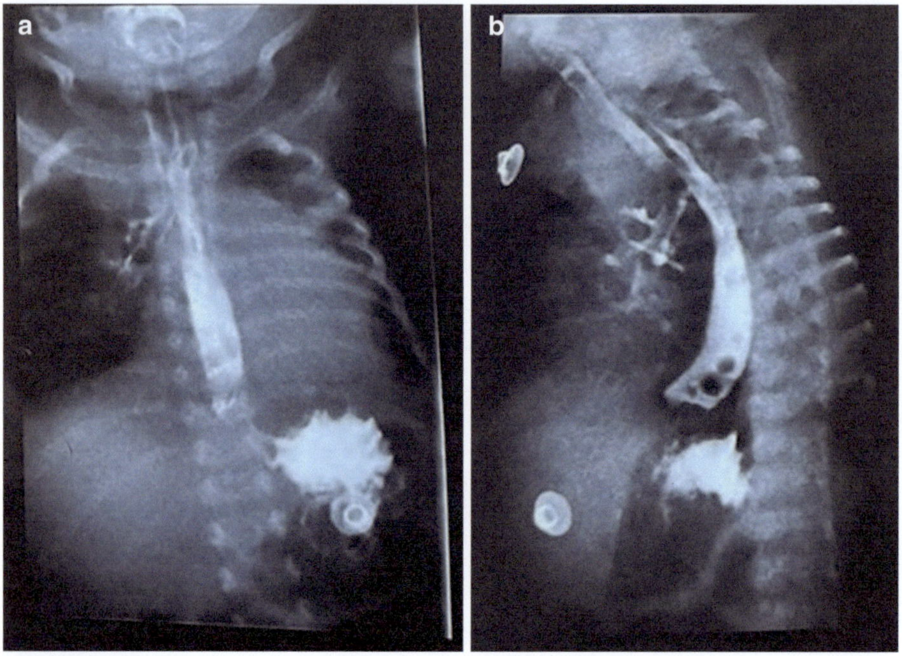

Fig. 15.30 Contrast esophagogram showing a recurrent TE fistula with dye going to the respiratory side (**a**) anterio-posterior view, (**b**) lateral view

Fig. 15.31 Intra-operative view showing the fistulous connection between the trachea and esophagus. This is at the original site of previous fistula ligation

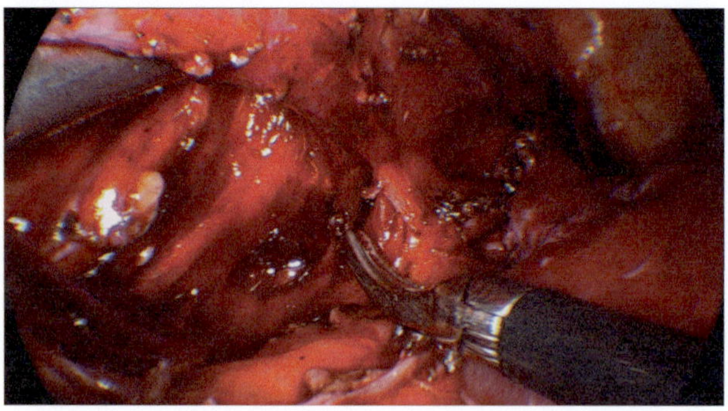

15.18 Conclusion

This chapter has presented a detailed pictographic account of the spectrum of TREAT procedure. The rest of the chapters supplement on detailed information on individual aspects of the procedure. All intra-operative pictures and imaging are original work of the author.

Suggested Reading

Kanojia R. Thoracoscopic repair of esophageal atresia (Unedited video). You Tube. 2020 April 16. https://youtu.be/CpZrisvHKWc?si=7kkufVt0O6YEx_h7.

Kanojia R. Upper pouch dissection in TREAT. You Tube. 2021 April 22. https://youtu.be/4U25E-1xKyw?si=tc0p2rz5PgTGkwcY.

Kanojia R. Thoracoscopic repair of esophageal atresia. 2017 Feb 23. You Tube. https://youtu.be/AhVactADAgg?si=bsqrZiX-mbeGWmOw.

Kanojia R. Radiology findings on pre op X-ray in Esophageal atresia with Tracheo-esophageal fistula. You Tube. 2020 March 25. https://youtu.be/En3HrdyGDC4?si=atOFnAqJX4MiQovA.

Kanojia R. Recurrent TE fistula after EA-TEF repair. You Tube. 2018 Feb 25. https://youtu.be/hdBY8pY4eh4?si=E2OSKuf4DO5HTMnZ.

Thoracoscopic repair of esophageal atresia with tracheo-esophageal atresia. (n.d.). SpringerLink. https://link.springer.com/video/10.1007/978-981-993624-3.

Operation Theatre Challenges, Integration, and Team Coordination During Neonatal Minimal-Access Procedure

16

Contents

Learning Objectives

1. Components and teams involved for TREAT
2. Role of individual teams
3. Interpersonal coordination and communication

16.1 Introduction

Neonatal minimal-access procedures are never a one-person task, and thoracoscopic repair of esophageal atresia is no exception. The procedure requires a team approach with several small groups working within the bigger team. A team is an identifiable set of two or more individuals working within a larger organizational context to

Supplementary Information The online version contains supplementary material available at https://doi.org/10.1007/978-981-97-5695-7_16.

R. P. Kanojia, *Thoracoscopic Repair of Esophageal Atresia*, https://doi.org/10.1007/978-981-97-5695-7_16

reach a common goal through specific interdependent roles and task boundaries [1]. The members of the team always have individual roles to play with a common goal. There is open communication with extensive flow of information with minutest of the details. This team system will always work as a soccer team where the quarter back is as important as the center forward. Even if the center forward scores a goal, he cannot be credited with the reason for winning because the people playing in the defendant's position have prevented conceding goals which made the team win.

There are several studies in surgery literature which have shown that improving teamwork with training and courses helps improve outcome with reduction in errors and mortality [2]. Success of thoracoscopic repair of esophageal atresia is declared only when the patient goes home without complications. The patient's journey from admission in surgical care unit to operation, postoperative care, and discharge to home is arduous and filled with high-risk situations and a real chance of mortality as the margin of error is very low with the patient. This is like the video game of obstacle course where the surgeon is making neonate jump through the loops and hoops of all the adverse factors. He moves through various levels along with the lead surgeon and his teammates. This works as a relay with handing over the baton from one stage to the other at various levels till final destination of discharge is reached.

This chapter lays out the structure of overall team organization and subgrouping to take care of the newborn. The discussions within the scope of this chapter are in general applicable to any organizational surgical setup.

16.2 Team Organization

There are four very important team subgroups within the larger departmental setup. Surgical team, pediatric anesthesia team, surgical intensivist team, and surgical nursing team. The neonate lies at the center of the Venn diagram of the area of expertise of these four teams (Fig. 16.1). These are analogous to four wheels of a car carrying the patient. This will not move anywhere if any one of the wheels is missing or not working efficiently. The outcome of the patient is heavily dependent on the interplay between these four teams. These teams will have a further sub-team within themselves with various members who will coordinate within the subgroup. The subsequent sections will describe these subgroup organizations and dynamics.

16.2.1 The Surgical Team

The surgeon is the lead and carries the final responsibility for the patient. He works in close coordination with his other surgical members. From the perspective of procedure intraoperatively, the most important person is the camera assistant. Assisting with thoracoscopic procedures has several challenges, and the assistant has to coordinate with the lead surgeon to complete the procedure in most efficient manner. The assistant should be trained in basics of laparoscopy and should be aware of the

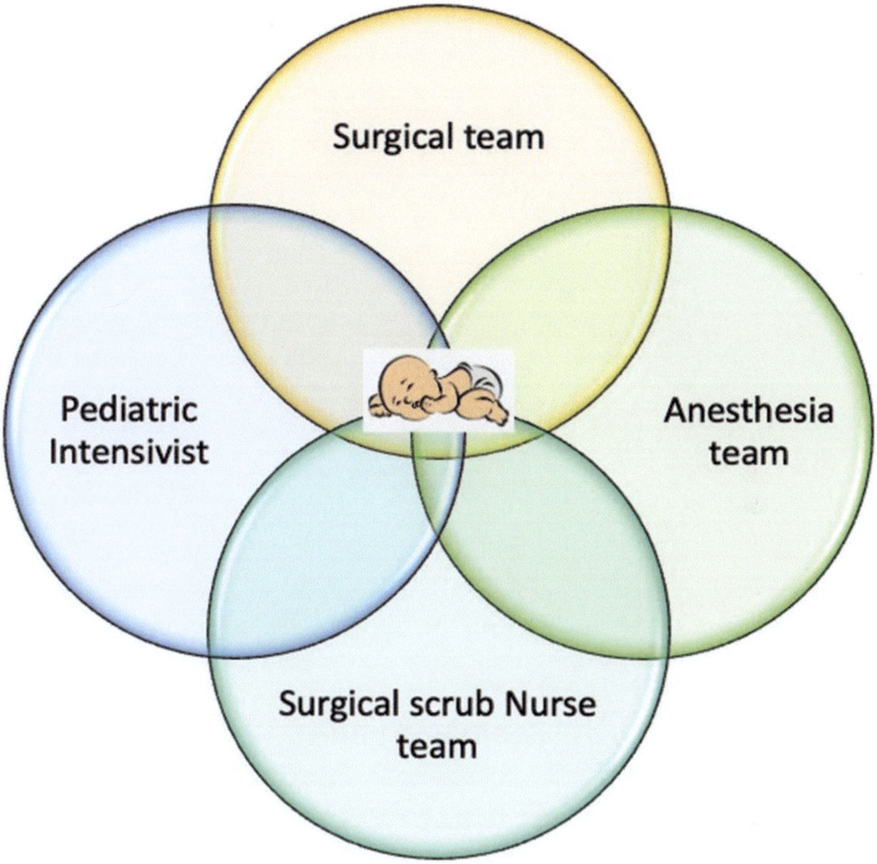

Fig. 16.1 Four essential components for neonatal minimal-access surgery. This is described as four wheels of a car analogy for conceptual understanding

optics. Below are the main challenges and the skill components required for the assistant which will increase the efficiency of the procedure. These components are depicted in Fig. 16.2 with the camera person at the center of the problems trying to overcome the challenges.

16.2.1.1 Moving Lung

The first and most important is the moving right lung. The lung control is discussed in other sections of this book. If this is efficiently done, the lung stays quiet, and the surgeon can complete the procedure. This however is not the case every time. There are cases where the lung is constantly moving and there is no clear view for the surgeon. There can be frequent desaturation, and the anesthetist will interrupt the surgeon to deflate the chest so that saturation can pick up. The camera assistant must find a way to give the best possible view with the lung jumping around. The best

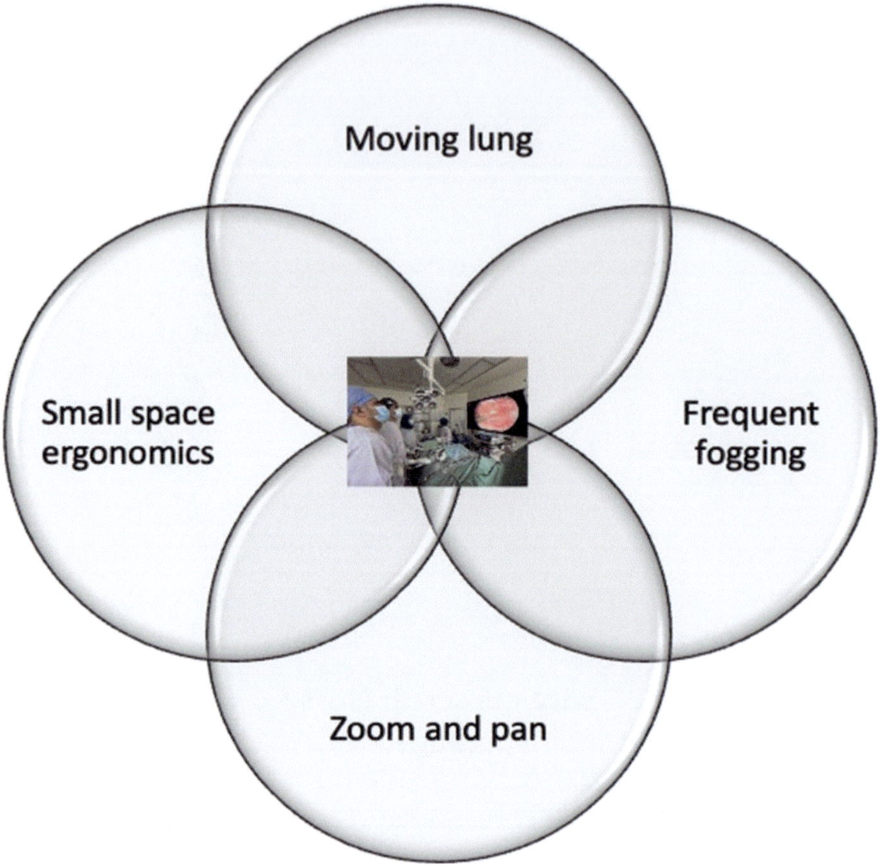

Fig. 16.2 Challenges for a camera assistant surgeon

way is to do this is by understanding the optics of a 30-degree telescope. The beveled tip of the telescope will give the ability to see past obstacles without making much of sideways movement at the level of camera hub. This is demonstrated by the video supplement cited below. If the light cable is tilted to 30–40 degrees without any change in the camera hub 12 o'clock position, a side-peeking view can be obtained through the obstacle which is directly in front of the tip of camera. As shown in the video, the number 2 on scale is not visible in neutral position of camera and light cable, but the number becomes visible once the bevel is made to angulate (Video 16.1).

This is an important optical principle in laparoscopic surgery and is applicable to all procedures irrespective of age and size. The lower lobe of the lung can be made to compress by the shaft of the telescope when the assistant is giving a close-up view by moving in towards the esophageal pouches.

16.2.1.2 Frequent Fogging

Fogging is a common problem during laparoscopy, and during thoracoscopy this can be a bigger problem because of the small working space, cold patient, and the lung surface frequently touching the tip of the telescope. This leads to frequent cycle of withdrawing the telescope—cleaning—re-entry. This will not only prolong the duration of procedure but also interrupt the surgeon's rhythm of dissection, and the longer this goes on, the higher will be the chances of errors. The best way to counteract this problem is to optimize the patient temperature and preheat the telescope tip in hot water. Vaporization and fogging are more on colder surfaces, so if the glass at the tip of the telescope is at the same or higher temperature to that of the chest cavity, fogging will not happen. Using cold CO_2 gas insufflation is another reason. In most of the modern setup, heated gas insufflators are available. They are expensive, and if not available then this must be tackled by methods described above. One of the ways to reduce the effect of cold gas is by attaching the gas connection to any port other than the optical port.

16.2.1.3 Zoom and Pan during the Procedure

Providing view on screen in laparoscopy is not a static procedure. The assistant must frequently move in and out to provide the best possible view for the intricate dissection done by the surgeon. Several steps like separating the upper pouch from the tracheal side require a crystal-clear view for the surgeon so that he appropriately finds a plane between the two organs. A millimeter deviation on either side can result in injury to the trachea or the esophagus. The assistant must understand this and must zoom in and out in the field of view depending on the requirement. In robotic surgery the surgeon has a major advantage as he can control the movement of the telescope and is not dependent on the assistant. This is not the case in laparoscopic surgery. Technical information required while zooming in and out of the field by the assistant is that most of the cameras available in current era are fixed focal length cameras. There may be a need to readjust the focus of the camera while zooming in and out by dynamically adjusting the focus ring on the camera hub. A good camera assistant will always identify the blurred out-of-focus view even before it comes on the screen. At present there is no autofocus telescope, and even in robotic surgery, the focus is to be adjusted manually. During suturing especially in a very small space, the zoom in and zoom out are even more important. When the surgeon is handling the needle inside the mediastinum, a wider view is needed so that the needle is safely handled around the vascular structures. When the tissue bite is taken with the needle during anastomosis, a close-up view is needed so that the bite includes the mucosa. Once the tissue bites are taken, the knot tying again requires a zoom out view. The assistant must understand this requirement and assist accordingly. In the author's experience the procedure time is significantly reduced if this concept is clearly understood by the assistant. A novice assistant will always wait for the instruction from the surgeon for moving in and out, increasing the procedure time.

16.2.1.4 Small Space Ergonomics

In neonatal surgery everything is small. The inside working space is small, and even the space outside the patient is limited for two surgeons, anesthetist, and scrub nurse with her trolley. There is barely any space for a second surgical assistant and is not needed also. Setup ergonomics are discussed in detail in Chap. 3. The challenge for the assistant is to position himself in this small space along with the surgeon. The important points to highlight here is that the assistant should not stand in perpendicular position to the line of SCOP. This will lead to more parallax movement and difficult hand-eye coordination.

16.2.2 The Anesthesia Team

The anesthesia team is the second most important component of the four-wheel drive approach of team organization. Maintaining the fragile neonate on a single lung with other comorbidities is not an easy task. This requires experience and understanding of neonatal physiology. Anesthesia and ventilation are discussed in detail in Chap. 4. From the perspective of team organization, the most important point to highlight here is the synchronization of ventilation with the surgeon and his instrument movements. It is extremely important that in the entire setup of displays available, there should be a monitor available in comfortable view of the anesthetist. Most often a senior anesthetist must sit through the entire procedure hand ventilating the neonate. If a good intraoperative view is provided to the anesthetist, he or she will be able to actively synchronize and take the surgeon through without much interruption and desaturation episodes. The main anesthetist is supplemented with assistant registrar and a technician. They will take care of other components of anesthesia work required during the procedure. The assistant anesthetist at a stage will insert infant feeding tube in the upper pouch. For this they must go under the drapes in a very awkward position. The requirements while doing this is to watch the upper pouch movements on screen while the assistant is pushing the tube and finer things like loss of pneumothorax pressure can occur when the upper pouch is opened and the eye on the tip of the feeding tube acts as a vent. To prevent this the feeding tube should be closed at the rear end. The assistant should also make sure that the feeding tube is not coiled in the mouth and the tip has reached the stomach. After completion of the procedure, the anesthesia team should be careful when the patient is handed over to them and neonate is repositioned supine and moved to upper end of the table. It goes without saying that all the lines including the trans-anastomotic tube should be careful preserved as they have the highest chance of dislodgement during this stage or later when the patient is shifted back to the intensive care unit.

16.2.3 Surgical Scrub Nurse Team

The coordination and work of the surgical scrub team start even before the surgeon starts operating. They have to coordinate in a clear manner and know the requirements of this complex surgical procedure. There should be a clear surgical know-how on what instruments and sutures will be needed. Prior discussion with the surgeon about the planning should be done. It is always desirable that the same scrub nurse assists so that she knows the requirements of the surgeon. But this may not be possible every time. A workaround this is to have a surgical book of preferences specific for a surgeon as well as a procedure. The scrub nurse who has assisted a thoracoscopic esophageal atresia repair should make a note of items used at the end of procedure and add to the preferences book. The next person can go through these notes and the list of items and prepare for the next case. This will greatly help even if he/she is assisting for the first time. There should be a floating nurse who assists from outside in providing items during the procedure.

In situations when procedure gets converted to open, the scrub nurse has to be ready with the open instruments trolley. On some occasions the conversion is done for complications like bleeding or air leak. In this situation time becomes a crucial factor. The scrub nurse with her floor assistant must be ready for a planned conversion or emergency conversion. The preparedness of the scrub nurse can make a big difference in the outcome of the patient.

An unaware nurse who is not prepared for the procedure will slow down the procedure increasing the anesthesia time for the neonate. A micromanagement for the instruments, sutures, and equipment by active scrub nurse goes a long way in increasing the team efficiency.

16.2.4 Neonatal Intensivist for Postoperative Care

Completion of the procedure is not equivalent to success. It was emphasized at the beginning of this chapter that success is declared only when the patient goes home with minimal or no morbidity. After the completion of procedure another battle with ventilation, sepsis and leak lie ahead of the neonate. Neonatal intensivist is crucial for this postoperative management which will involve ventilation, sepsis management, and other components of ICU care. No matter how good the surgeon has done his job, there is always a chance of mortality in postoperative period resulting from complications. Pulmonary management is a crucial component. Often these neonates are ventilated for weeks which may include high-frequency mode if needed. Many of these neonates have complex cardiac conditions and require management with ionotropic support and many other cardiac-specific drugs. Surgeons do not carry the expertise in this area, and the neonatologist is the best reliable team member who can handle these complexities. In the event of an anastomotic leak, either major or minor, the pulmonary morbidity is increased, and neonatologist must work in tandem with the surgeon to decide on various strategies. Sometimes decisions for re-exploration and diversion are taken after active discussion with the neonatologist. Thus, this fourth wheel of the car (analogy) is extremely crucial. Neonatologist is also like the last person in a 4 × 4 relay race which takes the neonate to the finishing line. A good intensive care setup with efficient neonatologist and his team will provide confidence to the surgeon for more and more difficult cases.

16.3 Interpersonal Coordination and Communication

The quality and efficiency of surgical procedure is greatly affected by coordination and effective communication. The team components described in this chapter are required to be technically skilled. Besides technical skills these members are required to be trained in some nontechnical skills which include interpersonal communication and use of shared knowledge. This is often ignored in the training of team members. Team training exercises are carried out in many hospitals to improve outcomes. One of the key elements required for effective interpersonal communication is familiarity of team members before the procedure. In a study by Yao Zhang et al., team familiarity significantly increased the efficiency of the procedure reducing the operating time significantly [2].

16.4 Conclusions

Neonatal minimal-access surgery is a team sport and not a solo performance of a single person. This chapter emphasizes the value of the four core team components, that is, surgeon, camera assistant, anesthetist, and neonatologist. This is seen as four wheels of a car analogy where all the four wheels must synchronize and run with same efficiency. The entire procedure slows down if any one of these four components is not working to its full potential.

References

1. Kozlowski SWJ, Bell BS. Work groups and teams in organizations. In: Borman WC, Ilgen DR, Klimoski RJ, editors. Handbook of psychology: industrial and organizational psychology, vol. 12. John Wiley & Sons, Inc.; 2003. p. 333–75. https://doi.org/10.1002/0471264385.wei1214.
2. Zhang Y, Zheng B. Familiarity of surgical teams: impact on laparoscopic procedure time. Am J Surg. 2022;224(5):1280–4. https://doi.org/10.1016/j.amjsurg.2022.06.002. Epub 2022 Jun 3

Suggested Reading

Holland AJ, McBride CA. Non-operative advances: what has happened in the last 50 years in paediatric surgery? J Paediatr Child Health. 2015;51(1):74–7. https://doi.org/10.1111/jpc.12461. Epub 2013 Dec 23

Manley BJ, Doyle LW, Davies MW, Davis PG. Fifty years in neonatology. J Paediatr Child Health. 2015;51(1):118–21. https://doi.org/10.1111/jpc.12798. Epub 2014 Dec 23

McBride CA, Holland AJ. Theatre of paediatric surgery. J Paediatr Child Health. 2015;51(1):98–102. https://doi.org/10.1111/jpc.12810.

Long-Term Musculoskeletal Implications of Neonatal Thoracotomy: Is Thoracoscopy Worth the Hype?

17

Contents

Learning Objectives

1. Evolutionary history of thoracotomy as a procedure in neonates
2. Anatomical structures likely to be injured during thoracotomy
3. Musculoskeletal complications due to neonatal thoracotomy
4. Literature review of musculoskeletal complications after thoracotomy
5. Thoracotomy vs thoracoscopy: where do we stand?

17.1 Introduction

Thoracotomy in a neonate is a major undertaking. Morbidity factors generated out of the chest opening in the short and long terms are numerous. In the short term, these are increased ventilation requirements, pain management, higher risk of wound infection, and resultant sepsis. In the long term, there are several musculoskeletal (MSK) issues less often discussed in the literature. Scoliosis, winging of the scapula, and chest asymmetry are long-term morbidities. Studies highlighting the

R. P. Kanojia, *Thoracoscopic Repair of Esophageal Atresia*,
https://doi.org/10.1007/978-981-97-5695-7_17

advantages of thoracoscopy over open repair often lead to the statements of higher incidence of musculoskeletal complications in the long term with thoracotomy. The incidence of MSK complications after thoracotomy is approximately 20–50% and varies over a wide range in different series. These series include not just esophageal atresia but other neonatal conditions as well requiring thoracotomy. With improving techniques of thoracotomy, these musculoskeletal complications have been minimized, especially with muscle-sparing and nerve-preserving incisions. This chapter outlines the possible musculoskeletal complications and examines the evidence in the literature about the long-term complications of neonatal thoracotomy and how much edge it provides in the short and long terms for neonates of esophageal atresia compared to TREAT.

17.2 Historical Evolution of Thoracotomy in Neonates for EA

The history of the evolution of surgical procedures for esophageal atresia is spread over the last 100 years. Richter M [1] did the first thoracotomy and attempted to ligate the fistula. He was successful, but the patient did not survive. The evolution of thoracotomy and surgical procedures after Richter has come a long way. History is discussed in detail in Chap. 1. What Richter did was essentially a posterior thoracotomy in a prone position with partial rib excision. He made a para-scapular incision (Fig. 17.1 marked A). Richter's thoracotomy was an extremely mutilating thoracotomy and contributed to the failures. Because of these failures, many surgeons, including William Ladd, altogether avoided thoracotomy in the newborn period [2]. The first successful repair via thoracotomy was done by Cameron Haight in 1941 [3]. He did a thoracotomy for repair and primary anastomosis. There is a detailed account of this first case [4]. He opened the chest with a left posterior-lateral thoracotomy with excision of segments of the 2nd–5th ribs to obtain exposure. His patients had all sorts of adventures in post-op with leaks and saliva coming out from chest tube. He even tried to place a trans-anastomotic tube, which came out of the chest wound defect. One can see that these thoracotomy methods were mutilating by today's standards and extremely extensive for the newborn. Later (after the year 2000), as neonatal surgery evolved, the description of the removal of rib segments is not found in the literature. In modern-day thoracotomy, the chest is opened with utmost care and diligence. The opening process is both muscle cutting and preserving depending on the surgeon's preference and the exposure required. More and more centers now prefer muscle-sparing thoracotomy. The nerve to latissimus dorsi is preserved by visualization. The rib retractors gently spread the ribs without any musculoskeletal damage. This is all done to minimize surgical trauma and prevent any morbidity related to thoracotomy.

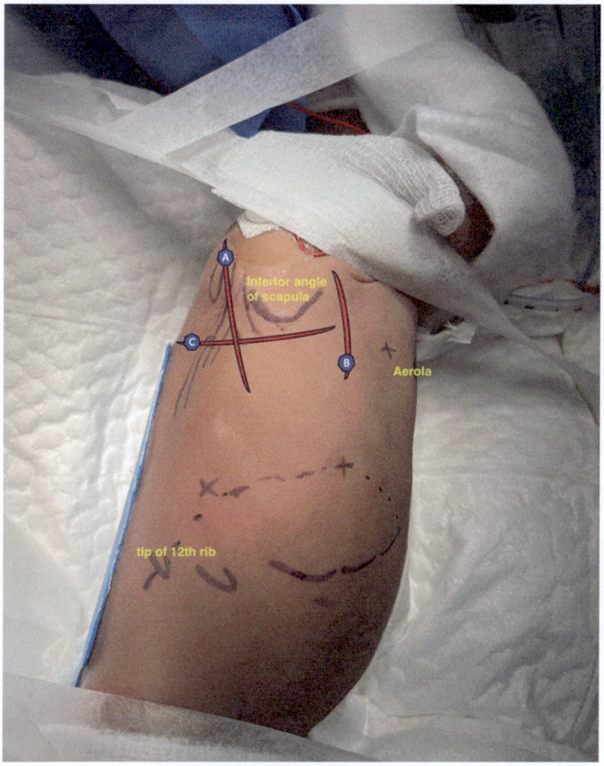

Fig. 17.1 Historical incisions for thoracotomy done in past A by Richter M, B is by Browne, C is conventional posterio-lateral thoracotomy incision

17.3 Anatomical Structures Likely to Be Injured during Thoracotomy

During thoracotomy, whether it is muscle sparing or muscle cutting, important musculoskeletal and neural structures can be injured. Injury to these structures is not always evident in the postoperative period in the neonate. The sequel is often evident years later when the child grows up. The cutting of chest wall muscles, serratus anterior, and latissimus dorsi is usually done in the thoracotomy incision. Apart from this, while cutting the muscles, the long thoracic nerve of the bell (LTNB) is most likely to be injured. LTNB, or posterior thoracic nerve, is the sole motor innervation to the serratus anterior with a root value of C567. The nerve runs over the chest wall very superficially in the midaxillary region (Fig. 17.2). This nerve is often visible while cutting the muscle and should be preserved. The nerve is so superficial

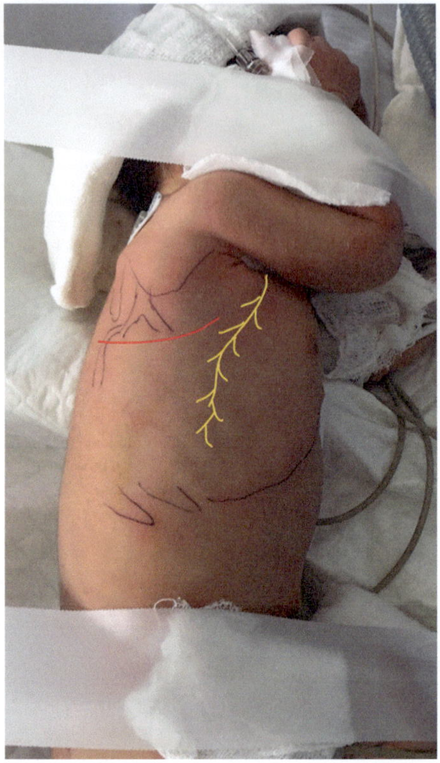

Fig. 17.2 Surface anatomy of long thoracic nerve

that it can even be injured during chest tube insertion. Injury to LTNB will result in the winging of the scapula [5]. The injury will only become apparent when the child starts walking and goes undetected in early life.

The thoracodorsal nerve is present as a neurovascular bundle and is a branch of the posterior cord of the brachial plexus with a root value of C7. This is a pure motor nerve to the latissimus dorsi, the climber's muscle of the human body. Partial or total division of these two important nerves and neurovascular bundle should be avoided, and the surgeon should be anatomically aware of it while opening the chest.

Besides this, there can be rib fusion due to the periosteal stripping of adjacent ribs of the open intercostal space [6]. The stripped areas, when approximated during the closure, will fuse by the periosteal reaction. This will result in chest asymmetry and, in the worst-case scenario, can cause secondary scoliosis even without any vertebral anomaly.

17.4 Possible Musculoskeletal Complications Due to Thoracotomy

Several MSK sequels can occur because of thoracotomy done in the neonatal period. These can be broadly divided into functional musculoskeletal complications and cosmetic complications. This section will discuss these two categories of sequelae and examine the incidence from the literature. For the sake of analysis, all neonates who have had thoracotomy for reasons other than esophageal atresia are also included, as the effect will be the same irrespective of the native condition.

17.4.1 Functional Musculoskeletal Complications

Major functional complications documented in the literature are scoliosis, limitation in range of motion in the ipsilateral shoulder joint, and winging of the scapula.

17.4.1.1 Scoliosis

Primary scoliosis can happen with esophageal atresia patients due to hemivertebrae or vertebral anomaly. Primary scoliosis can also happen due to neurological or muscular diseases like cerebral palsy. Secondary scoliosis can occur due to secondary effects of thoracotomy. Scoliosis is a three-dimensional spatial deformity of the spine with vertebral rotation on the axial plane, lateral curvature on the frontal plane, and sagittal deformity. Cobb's angle measures the severity of scoliosis [6]. An angle of less than 10° is acceptable and may not cause any problems. Scoliosis after thoracotomy in the neonatal period can happen due to multiple reasons. Rib fusion happening due to tight rib closure can cause scoliosis with concavity on the operated side. This can be more severe if the child has more than one exploration on the affected side. The complication of scoliosis is not evident until the age of 7 and increases with age. Specific radio-clinical follow-up is needed to detect scoliosis early in childhood. Surveillance is a must for redo thoracotomy patients. The treatment for such cases is variable. Mild cases can be managed conservatively. More severe cases will need braces for correction. Boston brace and Milwaukee brace are commonly prescribed for correcting the angle in younger children [7]. To protect spinal growth, surgical treatment is usually avoided. In cases of rib fusion, resection of the fused ribs may be required. Other surgical procedures required in extreme cases include vertebral fusion and vertical expandable prosthetic titanium rib placement with serial expansion done at regular intervals. In the majority of cases, the main predictive factor responsible is the division of muscles, excision of rib segments, and number of thoracotomies required in the neonatal period.

17.4.1.2 Ipsilateral Shoulder Abnormalities and Winging of Scapula

After scoliosis ipsilateral shoulder joint abnormalities are frequently encountered in follow-up. This includes restricted shoulder joint movement and, more commonly, winging of the scapula. This happens more with muscle-cutting approach where the muscles heal with some degree of fibrosis after re-suturing. There is some loss of muscle bulk in the recovery period. Since overhead shoulder movement is associated with rotation of the inferior angle of the scapula muscle, fibrosis in the latissimus dorsi muscle can cause partial fixing of the scapula, resulting in restriction in 360-degree shoulder joint movement. With muscle-cutting incisions, there can be injury to LTNB and thoracodorsal nerve, resulting in muscle atrophy, winging of the scapula, and chest wall asymmetry. Injury to the LTNB can not only be due to the actual division of the nerve but can also happen due to stretching and compression of the nerve during surgery for an extended period of time because of long surgery. Excessive use of electrocautery during the opening of the chest can also cause thermal damage to the nearby branches of the nerve to each of the serratus anterior digitations, resulting in partial denervation. This will cause winging of the scapula with unusual prominence of the medial border and inferior angle of the scapula. This is difficult to diagnose early in the neonatal period and becomes apparent only in long-term follow-up surveillance.

17.4.2 Cosmetic

Commonly possible cosmetic issues can be chest wall asymmetry, asymmetry of nipples, and chest wall deformity (pectus deformities). This is a result of rib approximation during the closure of thoracotomy and the division of muscles. During growth spurt, because there is some fibrosis in the muscles, there will be a differential growth in the bulk of the muscles. Also, because of the rib approximation, the intercostal space on the affected side will pull on for a long time while the rib cage is growing. The nipple to xiphisternal distance on the affected side will differ from the normal side, proving the asymmetry.

Breast Asymmetry in female patients is a very under-recognized cosmetic complication that can happen if the axillary tail of the breast gets caught in the incision cicatrix. With an anterior-lateral thoracotomy incision, there can be an injury to the breast bud, leading to maldevelopment later in life [8]. The chest wall asymmetry from rib fusion and scoliosis further accentuates the breast asymmetry in adult patients.

17.5 Literature Review of Musculoskeletal Complications after Thoracotomy in the Neonatal Period in Comparison to Thoracoscopy

The authors reviewed the literature for the incidence patterns for musculoskeletal issues in follow-up and how they compare with thoracotomy versus thoracoscopy. As described in an earlier section of this chapter about the evolution of thoracotomy methods, the methods of thoracotomy have changed from muscle cutting to muscle sparing. The incidence of complications with the older methods is very high, and including them will result in a biased heterogeneity of results. Hereafter, for the sake of uniformity, the review is restricted to the year 2000 and after. This is the same time frame when thoracoscopy started (1999—the first case of thoracoscopic repair) [9]. The series reported in the literature are tabulated and summarized below in Table 17.1.

Kengo Hattori et al. (2023) [10] presented a comparative cohort study between nine thoracoscopic and eight open repairs. Apart from other comparative parameters, long-term musculoskeletal outcomes were presented with 3/8 patients developing scoliosis and 4/8 patients developing chest wall asymmetry. In comparison, only one patient in the thoracoscopic group had chest wall asymmetry. The paper does not mention the mean follow-up duration of these patients. Also, there was no mention of the presence of any vertebral anomalies in these patients.

Unn Inger Møinichen et al. (2022) [11] evaluated 67 esophageal atresia adolescents (13–20 years) who had thoracotomy for repair. Significant scoliosis >20 deg.

Table 17.1 Summary of incidence patterns for musculoskeletal issues in follow-up patients of esophageal atresia and how they compare with thoracotomy versus thoracoscopy

S no.	Author (year)	No. of patients	Musculoskeletal complication rate	Comments
1.	**Kengo Hattori** et al. (2023) [10]	Comparative cohort study between nine thoracoscopic repair and eight open repair	3/8 patients developing scoliosis and 4/8 patients developing chest wall asymmetry. In comparison to this, only one patient in the thoracoscopic group had chest wall asymmetry	There was no mention of presence of any vertebral anomalies in these patients
2.	**Unn Inger Møinichen** et al. (2022) [11]	67 esophageal atresia adolescents (13–20 years)	12% (8 patients), mild scoliosis; severe scoliosis was present in 22% (15 patients) 22.3% overall rate of scoliosis	Of these 23 patients, 15 did not have any vertebral anomalies, and scoliosis was a consequence of thoracotomy
3.	**Divya G** et al. (2022) [12]	53 patients with thoracotomy for esophageal atresia and other thoracic conditions	19 patients (35.8%) had scoliosis	They concluded that tight chest wall closure is the main cause of the abnormalities in follow-up and should be avoided
4.	**Gustaf Drevin** et al. (2021) [13]	Systematic review and meta-analysis	Musculoskeletal complications are significantly higher in thoracotomy group (odds ratio 0.08 95% CI 0.01–0.58; $P = 0.0133$)	Only 2 studies out of 17 studies included in meta-analysis reported musculoskeletal complications
5.	**Nadia Safa** et al. (2021) [14]	104 patients who were younger than 14 years	39% (41/104) incidence of musculoskeletal abnormalities in follow-up	They concluded that division of serratus anterior muscle was a significant factor for developing MSK abnormalities in follow-up in esophageal atresia patients

(continued)

Table 17.1 (continued)

S no.	Author (year)	No. of patients	Musculoskeletal complication rate	Comments
6.	**Prabal R Mishra et al**. (2020) [15]	1338 patients' data was analyzed	Overall 268 (20%) had scoliosis. After excluding the congenital musculoskeletal anomalies, there was a 13% incidence of scoliosis due to thoracotomy	Independent risk factors for scoliosis were repeated thoracotomies, rib fusion, rib resection, and pleural fibrosis
7.	**Hiroomi Okuyama** et al. (2017) [16]	69 long-term patients of esophageal atresia with age >15	Musculoskeletal deformity in 59% (40/69) of cases	Limitation of this study is that there was no mention of rate of vertebral anomalies in the studied cohort
8.	**Panda SS** et al. (2013) [8]	52 patients less than 12 years of age	Winging of scapula in 5.7% (3/52), scoliosis with Cobb's angle >10 deg. in 1.9% (1/52)	This was relatively less as compared to the other series reported and summarized above
9.	**Taiwo A et al.** (2009) [17]	62 patients with a mean follow-up duration of 3.8 years. Thoracoscopy was done in 34/62 patients, and thoracotomy was done in 28/62 patients	54% of thoracotomy patients had scoliosis as compared to 10% thoracoscopy group	Indications for thoracic procedures were mixed including causes other than esophageal atresia

Cobb's angle was present in 12% (8 patients), and mild scoliosis (10–19 deg) was present in 22% (15 patients). Of these 23 patients, 15 had no vertebral anomalies, and scoliosis was a consequence of thoracotomy. The final incidence of isolated scoliosis was 22.3% in this series. There was atrophy of the right pectoralis muscle in more than two-thirds of patients. Apart from scoliosis, they measured muscle strength and functional exercise capacity and assessed motor skills. They concluded that exercise capacity in young EA patients is significantly lower due to scoliosis and other MSK abnormalities.

Divya G et al. (2022) [12] studied 53 patients who had undergone neonatal thoracotomy for esophageal atresia and other thoracic conditions requiring thoracotomy. They reported that 19 patients (35.8%) had scoliosis or other skeletal abnormality. They concluded that tight chest wall closure is the leading cause of the follow-up abnormalities and should be avoided.

Gustaf Drevin et al. (2021) [13] presented a systematic review and meta-analysis comparing thoracotomy and thoracoscopy for esophageal atresia and compared many parameters for outcome analysis. They reported that the musculoskeletal complications are significantly higher in thoracotomy group (odds ratio 0.08 95% CI 0.01–0.58; $P = 0.0133$). Only two studies out of 17 included in the meta-analysis reported musculoskeletal complications.

Nadia Safa et al. (2021) [14] studied a cohort of 104 patients who were younger than 14 years. The median follow-up duration was 10.8 years. The cohort included in this study did not have any vertebral anomaly or other congenital predisposition for musculoskeletal issues. They reported 39% (41/104) of musculoskeletal abnormalities in follow-up. Of these 41 patients, winging of the scapula was present in 24 (23%), scoliosis in 17 (16%), and chest wall anomalies in 15 (14%) of patients. They concluded that the division of the serratus anterior muscle was a significant factor for developing MSK abnormalities in follow-up in esophageal atresia patients.

Prabal R Mishra et al. (2020) [15] presented a systematic review with 14 studies analyzed. Total no of 1338 patients' data was analyzed and 268 (20%) had scoliosis. After excluding the congenital musculoskeletal anomalies there was a 13% incidence of scoliosis due to thoracotomy. Independent risk factors for scoliosis were repeated thoracotomies, rib fusion, rib resection, and pleural fibrosis.

Hiroomi Okuyama et al. (2017) [16] analyzed 69 long-term patients of esophageal atresia with age > 15 years. He reported musculoskeletal deformity in 59% (40/69) of cases. Of these 40 patients, 37% (25/68) had scoliosis, and 12% (8/68) had chest wall deformity. And 26% (18/68) had elevated scapula. This rate of musculoskeletal complications is very high as compared to other series. One limitation of this study is that there was no mention of the rate of vertebral anomalies in the studied cohort.

Panda SS et al. (2013) [8] did a cross-sectional analysis of all patients with thoracotomy for esophageal atresia or other conditions. Recruited patients were less than 12 years old and had a minimum of 2 years of follow-up. They studied 52 patients; there was winging of the scapula in 5.7% (3/52), scoliosis with Cobb's angle >10 deg. in 1.9% (1/52). This was relatively less as compared to the other series reported and summarized above.

Taiwo A et al. (2009) [17] studied neonatal thoracotomy outcomes in 62 patients with a mean follow-up duration of 3.8 years. The indications of thoracotomy were mixed. Thoracoscopy was done in 34/62 patients, and thoracotomy was done in 28/62 patients. The two groups were compared for complications related to MSK. They reported that 54% of thoracotomy patients had scoliosis compared to 10% of the thoracoscopy group.

Several other studies reported before 2000 document even higher rates of musculoskeletal complications. Robert P reported the first such study during 1980 [18]. Nine out of 18 patients had severe scoliosis. He concluded that rib resection is a major reason for musculoskeletal deformity.

17.6 Thoracotomy Vs Thoracoscopy: Where Do we Stand?

After the in-depth literature review, where do we stand on comparing thoracotomy and thoracoscopy? With the data presented, the incidence of musculoskeletal complications ranges from 20% to 50% in the series quoted above. We have included studies after 2000 so that a bias due to primitive methods of thoracotomy is excluded. Studies before the year 2000 report musculoskeletal complications of >60% due to the practice of rib excision and muscle-cutting incisions. It must be emphasized that many musculoskeletal complications in follow-up are under-recognized and active surveillance is needed after esophageal atresia repair. Patients are often diagnosed after puberty, so they may not be referred to the parent pediatric surgery team. Orthopedics more commonly see them, and hence, the long-term complications data available for pediatric surgeons may be under-notified.

Esophageal atresia repair by thoracoscopy is a difficult procedure with a long learning curve. Even if a skilled minimal-access surgeon is available, not every center has the complete setup, including an expert neonatal anesthetist and NICU setup. Does the data presented above mean that thoracotomy, which is the gold standard for esophageal atresia repair, is a procedure with high long-term complications? The answer is yes if the technique of thoracotomy is terrible. The answer is no if the method of opening the thorax is carried out with utmost diligence, preserving the musculature and the superficial nerves, and at the same time, closure is done without rib fusion. Beginner surgeons should always learn thoracotomy from expert mentors and should always have long-term complications at the back of their minds while running a knife over a delicate newborn.

TREAT is a 25-year-old procedure, and with the available follow-up studies, the long-term musculoskeletal complications are significantly less in these patients (less than 10%). All the short-term and long-term complications due to the opening of the chest in a newborn are avoided. Definitely, this gives an advantage in terms of faster recovery and fewer long-term complications. However, the surgeon should only push for thoracoscopy in the presence of expertise and the required setup. The gold standard for treatment of esophageal atresia is uncomplicated primary anastomosis. Whether this is achieved by thoracotomy or thoracoscopy depends on individual preference and available setup. Both methods should give an expectant outcome of full recovery.

References

1. Richter H. Congenital atresia of the oesophagus: an operation designed for its cure. Surg Gynecol Obstet. 1913;17:397–402.
2. Ladd WE. The surgical treatment of esophageal atresia and tracheoesophageal fistulas. N Engl J Med. 1944;230(21):625–37.
3. Haight C. Some observations on esophageal atresias and tracheoesophageal fistulas of congenital origin. J Thorac Surg. 1957;34(2):141–72.
4. Langston HT. The first successful total repair of congenital atresia of the esophagus with tracheoesophageal fistula. Ann Thorac Surg. 1984;38(1):72–4.
5. Bastard F, Bonnard A, Rousseau V, Gelas T, Michaud L, Irtan S, et al. Thoracic skeletal anomalies following surgical treatment of esophageal atresia. Lessons from a national cohort. J Pediatr Surg. 2018;53(4):605–9.
6. Popescu D, Merhi DA, Amellal O. Scoliosis caused by rib fusion after thoracotomy for esophageal atresia: a case report and surgical approach. J Orthop Case Rep. 2024;14(1):125–30.
7. Grivas TB, Negrini S, Aubin CE, Aulisa AG, De Mauroy JC, Donzelli S, et al. Nonoperative management of adolescent idiopathic scoliosis (AIS) using braces. Prosthetics Orthot Int. 2022;46(4):383–91.

8. Panda SS, Agarwala S, Bhatnagar V, Kabra SK, Jayaswal A, Bhalla AS. A survey of musculoskeletal and aesthetic abnormalities after thoracotomy in pediatric patients. J Indian Assoc Pediatr Surg. 2013;18(4):136–42.
9. Lobe TE, Rothenberg S, Waldschmidt J, Stroedter L. Thoracoscopic repair of esophageal atresia in an infant: a surgical first. Pediatr Endosurg Innov Tech. 1999;3(3):141–8.
10. Hattori K, Kawashima H, Ishimaru T, Yanagida Y, Miyake K, Iguchi M, Oiki H, Maeda S, Ihara Y. Musculoskeletal deformities after thoracoscopic versus conventional open repair for esophageal atresia. Asian J Surg. 2024;47(2):968–2
11. Moinichen UI, Mikkelsen A, Gunderson R, Kibsgard TJ, Morkrid L, IJsselstijn H, et al. New insights in the prevalence of scoliosis and musculoskeletal asymmetries in adolescents with esophageal atresia. J Pediatr Surg. 2023;58(3):412–9.
12. Divya G, Kundal VK, Debnath PR, Addagatla RS, Garbhapu AK, Saha AK, et al. Musculoskeletal and esthetic complications after neonatal thoracotomy: revisited. J Indian Assoc Pediatr Surg. 2022;27(3):293–6.
13. Drevin G, Andersson B, Svensson JF. Thoracoscopy or thoracotomy for esophageal atresia: a systematic review and meta-analysis. Ann Surg. 2021;274(6):945–53.
14. Safa N, Wei S, Saran N, Guadagno E, Laberge JM, Emil S. Musculoskeletal deformities after thoracic surgery in children: an observational long-term follow-up study. J Pediatr Surg. 2021;56(1):136–41.
15. Mishra PR, Tinawi GK, Stringer MD. Scoliosis after thoracotomy repair of esophageal atresia: a systematic review. Pediatr Surg Int. 2020;36(7):755–61.
16. Okuyama H, Tazuke Y, Uenoa T, Yamanaka H, Takama Y, Saka R, et al. Long-term morbidity in adolescents and young adults with surgically treated esophageal atresia. Surg Today. 2017;47(7):872–6.
17. Lawal TA, Gosemann JH, Kuebler JF, Gluer S, Ure BM. Thoracoscopy versus thoracotomy improves midterm musculoskeletal status and cosmesis in infants and children. Ann Thorac Surg. 2009;87(1):224–8.
18. Durning RP, Scoles PV, Fox OD. Scoliosis after thoracotomy in tracheoesophageal fistula patients. A follow-up study. J Bone Joint Surg Am. 1980;62(7):1156–9.

MIX
Papier aus verantwortungsvollen Quellen
Paper from responsible sources
FSC® C105338

If you have any concerns about our products,
you can contact us on
ProductSafety@springernature.com

In case Publisher is established outside the EU,
the EU authorized representative is:
Springer Nature Customer Service Center GmbH
Europaplatz 3, 69115 Heidelberg, Germany

Printed by Libri Plureos GmbH
in Hamburg, Germany